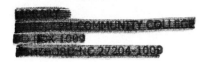

SPIRITUALITY IN NURSING

The Challenges of Complexity

Third Edition

Barbara Stevens Barnum, RN, PhD, is a noted presence in nursing education, the author of twelve books (five published by Springer), many with numerous additional editions, with chapters appearing in numerous other titles, and many peer-reviewed articles. She has served as Editor of *Nursing Leadership Forum* (Springer), and Editor of *Nursing & Health Care* (the previous incarnation of the National League for Nursing's *Nursing Education Perspectives*). Currently, she is a consultant, psychotherapist, and (part-time faculty) periodic lecturer at NYU, Nursing. Previous positions include Director, Division of Health Services, Sciences and Education, Teachers College, New York, where she also held the Stewart Chair, and chair in the Department of Nursing Education. She was a consultant at the Columbia-Presbyterian Medical Center, New York, with a prior academic position as professor, Nursing Administration, College of Nursing, the University of Illinois, Chicago. A fellow of the American Academy of Nursing, Dr. Barnum has done extensive national and international consultation, including an 8-year term as consultant to the Air Force Surgeon General. Dr. Barnum presents workshops in areas of complementary medicine and spirituality nationwide.

Spirituality in Nursing

The Challenges of Complexity

Third Edition

BARBARA STEVENS BARNUM, RN, PhD

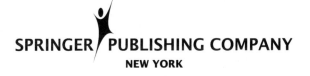

SPRINGER PUBLISHING COMPANY
NEW YORK

Springer Publishing Company, LLC
11 West 42nd Street
New York, NY 10036
www.springerpub.com

Acquisitions Editor: Allan Graubard
Project Editor: Peter Rocheleau
Project Manager: Ragavia Ramakrishnan
Cover Design: Mimi Flow
Composition: S4Carlisle Publishing Services

ISBN: 978-0-8261-0583-7
E-book ISBN: 978-0-8261-0584-4

10 11 12 13/ 5 4 3 2 1

The author and the publisher of this Work have made every effort to use sources believed to be reliable to provide information that is accurate and compatible with the standards generally accepted at the time of publication. Because medical science is continually advancing, our knowledge base continues to expand. Therefore, as new information becomes available, changes in procedures become necessary. We recommend that the reader always consult current research and specific institutional policies before performing any clinical procedure. The author and publisher shall not be liable for any special, consequential, or exemplary damages resulting, in whole or in part, from the readers' use of, or reliance on, the information contained in this book. The publisher has no responsibility for the persistence or accuracy of URLs for external or third-party Internet Web sites referred to in this publication and does not guarantee that any content on such Web sites is, or will remain, accurate or appropriate.

Library of Congress Cataloging-in-Publication Data

Barnum, Barbara Stevens.
  Spirituality in nursing: the challenges of complexity / Barbara Stevens
Barnum.—3rd ed.
      p.; cm.
  Includes bibliographical references and index.
  ISBN 978-0-8261-0583-7—ISBN 978-0-8261-0584-4 (e-book)
  1. Nursing—Religious aspects.   2. Nursing—Philosophy.   3. Nursing—Psychological
aspects.   4. Spirituality. I. Title.
  [DNLM: 1. Nurse-Patient Relations.   2. Spirituality.   3. Philosophy, Nursing.
4. Religion and Medicine. WY 87 B263s 2010]
  RT85.2.B37 2010
  610.7301—dc22

                                                                      2010021860

Printed in the United States of America by the Hamilton Printing Company

To my daughter, Lauren Stevens

Contents

Preface

Starting afresh is essential in just about anything these days. Too much is rote, too much old hat, too much just doesn't work as it should or could be, given better circumstances. The subject of spirituality in nursing is no different. So when I considered a new edition, I also considered what issues had stumped or frustrated me over the years.

What are the real issues that nurses confront when dealing with patients' spiritual problems or even when dealing with their own spiritual problems?

This means that the present edition is more about thinking than referencing, more about identifying problems than sticking to expected topics. It also means that my own opinions (and prejudices) are present in some chapters. And finally, from my perspective, it means that this edition was much more interesting and, yes, more fun to write. I hope you will find it more interesting and more fun to read.

The *Introduction* that immediately follows this preface will briefly survey what I found, and still find, problematic. The rest of the book will tell you why these problems existed then and exist today, and what can (or can't) be done about them.

I might add one observation that underlies the relationship between nursing and spirituality in every era. And here's the pathway: Modern nursing started out with an important relationship. Spirituality was closely linked to nursing's definition as *an art and a science.*

As practitioners of nursing worried about becoming professional and academic, however, its artistry weakened, with much of it discarded, in fact, including the focus on spirituality. This tendency was reinforced by accreditors who evaluated performance by nurses and schools of nursing in terms of "outcome objectives." As spiritual goals are complex, they simply do not fit within specified outcomes.

But now the tables have turned. There is a thrust to return spirituality to its earlier preeminence in nursing. Yet how that's done also can be problematic, making the nurse's role more difficult. My point is that our actions have always been motivated by social changes rather than considering what these changes really mean for nurses, nursing, and the clients we serve. Stay tuned to the book to find my responses to these often tricky situations.

One other issue: My editor thinks you should know who I am—something that I didn't worry about in prior editions. I wanted the content of the book to speak for itself. That, of course, is silly, and he's right—something I rarely admit. So here's a brief synopsis of how I've spent my career in nursing—so far!

I began my nursing education in one of the very early associate of arts of nursing programs. This served me very well because I always enjoyed a little conflict. Sadly, whatever age you are, you know the eternal and unresolved arguments between associate degree nursing programs and bachelor's programs. The beginning of my nursing in an associate degree program assured me that many nurse leaders of the time would forever think of me as being problematic. I became more problematic by completing a master's degree in educational administration and a doctorate at the University of Chicago in philosophy and education.

I began my nursing career in Labor and Delivery in St. Petersburg, Florida, at the then named Mound Park Hospital. This was a position that I loved dearly. But then I made a visit to a friend in Chicago and somehow ended up teaching Fundamentals of Nursing at Augustana Hospital and Health Care Center. Somehow, my career has been more serendipity than planning. Next, I found myself heading that school, getting it ready to convert to a baccalaureate program. Strangely, that didn't happen once I left and turned the position over to someone more educationally qualified to head a baccalaureate program.

Meanwhile, I had a fascinating alternate career as Director of Nursing Service at the same institution. And then somehow I moved on to head a program in Nursing Administration at the University of Illinois. This was at a time when nursing administration was disdained by many clinical faculty—which made it just my sort of assignment. And by then I had a doctorate, which meant I could overcome many previous frustrations. It was an era when very few doctorates were available in nursing, so my degree in another field was no obstacle then.

From there, Teachers College, Columbia University, wooed me to its nursing program (which I headed along with the other health programs there). I retired from that position with an apparent incapacity to stay indolent, returning to Columbia in two other roles, including one at the uptown nursing program of Columbia. While Teachers College, Columbia University, focused on preparing nursing teachers and administrators, the uptown School of Nursing, Columbia University, focused on preparing clinicians.

In between these ventures, I twice served as an editor of a nursing journal—another job I truly loved. Nursing has been good to me in always providing new interests. It's wonderful to be able to be a vagabond, always doing different things, in a profession with such diversity.

After my last retirement from Columbia, I felt an urge for something different (surprise!) and studied psychoanalysis for nearly 4 years, this after teaching mostly nursing administration, nursing theory, and doctoral dissertation courses. Yes, a vagabond.

Introduction

I approached this third edition of *Spirituality in Nursing* from a different perspective. Primarily, I tried to base each chapter on a question or series of questions concerning a given topic. These were questions that had puzzled me and, on the whole, had given the nursing profession problems. What, for example, do we do about the zealously religious, but spiritually immature, nurse who thinks she has answers for every patient? How do we research an evanescent subject like spirituality?

The chapter topics are simply those on which I've stubbed my toes over the years. The reader who is looking for answers may be frustrated with this book because some chapters simply discover more questions than answers. For example, what happens when a profession expects nurses to deal with patients' spiritual problems but gives the nurses absolutely no education from which to do that? Theologians and philosophers spend lifetimes unraveling spiritual challenges, yet nurses are expected to deal with a patient's most serious spiritual problems with no education for it—and in a flash, between tending to other tasks for life-impairing injuries or disease states. No, there are no easy answers for situations like this—just more questions.

Then there is the challenge of the very topic of spirituality. Spirituality may be different for every human being. How do we handle a subject matter like that? And how do we convert it into meaningful suggestions for nursing action? Nevertheless, I hope that the reader will come away with a sense of the depth of the problems that arise when nurses deal with spirituality.

There is no end to the problems. I remember when I was a young nurse in a Veteran's Administration Hospital, and a young quadraplegic patient told me that a nurse had said to him, "You killed people in war, and now look what God has done to punish you." Now what on earth could I have said to take the sting out of that comment? I still remember this incident more than 50 years after it happened. Can I imagine how long that comment stayed with the patient? What could I possibly have responded that would have had equal impact on his thoughts? Again, just questions.

Then there are the internal thoughts that matter as much as the responses one makes. I remember a mob hit man who was so grateful to me that he said, "Just name him; for you, I'll kill whoever you want." I knew how carefully the mob controlled their psychopathic hit men (of which he clearly was one). Mob psychopaths don't have the option of picking their own targets—not if they want to live. The definition of a psychopath kept spinning in my brain—someone with no real feelings. How did I justify that definition with those weird but apparently heartfelt words from a man who supposedly had no heart? What problems are psychological, what ones are spiritual? Need I add that this was an offer I never accepted.

My first experience with a patient just returning from a near-death experience: her joy as she began to describe her journey. And then the puzzled and distraught expression on her face when her physician said, "Don't pay any attention to that. You were just hallucinating." Every nurse who stays in the profession long enough will have his or her own list of spiritual memories that nick at the back of the mind.

Almost every chapter in this book raises a puzzling question. Is spirituality a natural part of growth and development? If so, what happens when the nurse is more immature than the patient?

Or spirituality and the brain: Is spirituality all chemistry and genes? True, we keep finding more connections, but what does that mean? Is spirituality no different than red hair? And is spirituality genetic?

Or spirituality and healing: Should nursing make an investment in healing, a domain it cannot own? Ministers have used laying-on-of-hands for centuries. Does spirituality enter into healing? Or is there a physiological explanation?

What are the major challenges facing the nurse who wants to incorporate spiritual care in practice? Can we draw some conclusions for the future of nursing and spirituality?

One thing this book will *not* deal with is the ultimate nature of reality. Yet we know that some disciplines are invested in a materialistic notion of the world that basically denies the reality of things spiritual. This belief, for example, still dominates in the field of psychoanalysis. But we will not worry about what is *real*, we will only concern ourselves with what is *believed* to be real by either the nurse or the patient. We will deal with the patient's (and nurse's) convictions and how they influence their lives.

We are seeing a resurgence of interest in spirituality in nursing today—perhaps because other aspects of our practice look so bleak. Nurses feel overworked, overstressed, and often helpless to improve their work situation. Yet at a time when at least some nurses feel spiritually bankrupt, accreditors and evaluators of all sorts are adding spiritually related tasks to lists of required nursing functions. Does this make sense? And why is it happening now?

Perhaps we are looking in the wrong direction. Perhaps nurses have more spiritual needs than most patients. Can the frustration of the nurse's job have raised spiritual issues on his or her part?

Further, in hospital facilities, patients are sicker and more likely to voice spiritual needs. Yet patients are also discharged rapidly, making it less likely that their spiritual problems will be solved during a quick hospital stay. Spiritual problems are not easily solved; they can't be rapidly bandaged and forgotten.

This book, then, is mostly about spiritual issues and challenges that arise in the health care setting. Many of the problems raised are simply pragmatic, yet most are intellectual as well.

Spiritual questions posed in this book include but are not limited to the following.

A. For the practicing nurse:
   1. What should the nurse do if he or she feels unprepared for spiritual counseling?
   2. How can a nurse decide when to handle a spiritual problem and when to call in a spiritual professional?
B. For the patient:
   1. How does the patient protect his spiritual privacy?
   2. How can the patient ensure that the staff protects his spiritual privacy?
   3. The patient may be more spiritually sophisticated than the nurse. How does he handle the nurse who is trying to perform an inappropriate spiritual intervention?
C. For the teacher in schools or in-service education:
   1. On one level, spirituality can't be taught as much as caught. How then is it conveyed to nurses?
   2. What are the best teaching methods to ensure inculcation of spiritual values in students?
D. For the nurse manager:
   1. Spirituality involves different professions (religious ministries, schools of philosophy), and the nurse may not be as knowledgeable as he or she thinks. How do we handle the nurse's lack of sophistication and misperceptions?
   2. Some nurses wish to proselytize their own religion. How can this practice be stopped?
   3. Some nurses are subjected to nursing diagnostic guidelines that force spiritual evaluations and therapy upon them. These formulas almost always give health goals priority over spiritual goals. What do we do when nurses are encouraged to produce comfort at all cost?

4. The patient may be more spiritually sophisticated than the nurse who thinks he or she should determine the other's spiritual direction. How can we deal with this imbalance?
5. What is to be done when either the patient or the nurse seeks to place blame or guilt for circumstances? What spiritual issues are raised with such judgments? And how do we stop this dangerous practice?

This book may not present all the answers to these dilemmas, but hopefully, the reader will be more aware of the problems and the issues when he or she finishes reading this book.

SPIRITUALITY IN NURSING

The Challenges of Complexity

Third Edition

CHAPTER 1

Spiritual Versus Religious Orientations

Spirituality and religion are often blended as if they were one. However, it is important for nurses to recognize the differences between the two. True, for some people spirituality is closely tied to their religion, but that's not true in everyone's case. Some people practice a religion for social, political, or cultural reasons without deriving much spiritual value from it. Alternately, some people are highly spiritual without following a religion at all.

How are religion and spirituality different from each other? What is the advantage of treating them separately? When does it matter? Should one or both be the target for nursing evaluation and/or actions?

Before we can discuss the interface between spirituality and religion, these two concepts need to be differentiated. Moreover, the reader should bear in mind that the focus of this book is spirituality. As seen in Chapter 5, it isn't always possible to give a precise operational definition for spirituality. By its very nature, spirituality presents a challenge. It is difficult to pin down a concept that is different for everyone. In an era when everything about nursing has been reduced to very concrete care objectives, some readers will have trouble with this degree of ambiguity.

SPIRITUALITY

In looking for a good definition of *spirituality*, I found that William James's (1997) definition came closer to my conception than any other author's. James, of course, didn't write at the time of the copyright listed above. Indeed, his classic book (a compilation of his lectures on religion at the University of Edinburgh) was first published in 1902, and had been reprinted numerous times. Yet no one surpasses James in capturing the essence of spirituality.

Ironically, the title of the book in which these lectures appear is *The Varieties of Religious Experience*.

I say ironically because James really is interested in spirituality, rather than religion. Yet it is not surprising that he speaks of religion instead because these lectures were the product of his appointment at the University of Edinburgh as Gifford Lecturer on Natural Religion. James, himself, had credentials in psychology; he was not a theologian.

After his appointment, James quickly dissected religion to isolate the part that he wished to examine. First, he eliminated "the systematic theology and ideas about the gods themselves" (p. 41). He then stated what *religion* would mean for him, that is: "the feelings, acts, and experiences of individual men in their solitude, so far as they apprehend themselves to stand in relation to whatever they may consider the divine" (p. 42). James is clear that the *divine* may be a concrete deity or not (p. 45). He is also clear that his notion of what matters in a religion is that which is experienced directly, not what is discussed philosophically.

Hence, his first act was to slice up religion, indicating the aspect that held his attention. In addition, that slice is exactly what I mean by spirituality. James then noted that "the personal religion will prove itself more fundamental than either theology or ecclesiasticism" (p. 42). James further specified this component by noting that, although it may bring happiness, the happiness comes with a sense of solemnity, parted off from what he calls *mere animal happiness*.

One thing I would emphasize in labeling James' description as spirituality is that a person can meet this definition without following a religion at all—a comment James could only make delicately as Gifford Lecturer on Natural Religion.

James is not the only one to capture this element as the most important one in religion. Theologian Henri Nouwen (1972), in reaching for the characteristics required by effective ministers, sets as prerequisite the condition that all ministers must "enter ourselves first of all into the center of our existence and become familiar with the complexities of our inner lives" (p. 38). And that "only he who is able to articulate his own experience can offer himself to others as a source of clarification" (p. 38).

James and Nouwen, then, represent those reaching for that slice of being that captures the inner experience of divinity. I label this element as spirituality and, as James did, take it to mean the feelings, acts, and experiences of people as they apprehend themselves in relation to whatever they may consider the divine, that is, in relation to what is most meaningful to them from the larger, solemn focus on reality as they comprehend it.

How else might we define spirituality? Spirituality has about it a sense of the transcendent. It deals with those values that reach beyond the material world and its self-serving goals. These are the values not merely espoused but deeply felt within by humans. Of course, these same feelings may exist as part of religion. Spirituality, then, is experiential, existential, and touches the inner core of each human being, where he or she most truly lives.

RELIGION

In contrast to spirituality (which is highly personal), religion, no matter what its origin, evolves as a social institution. It is an organization that binds people together in many ways. Part of the binding comes from its shared beliefs, part from communal membership, and part from shared rituals. Among its parts, for many members, will also be that component we call spirituality.

By the time a religion is formulated and organized, its beliefs and customs are usually somewhat or even greatly distorted from the teachings of the religion's founder. Organized religions usually begin in the vision of a mystic, one who draws his inspiration and insight from an intense and personal relationship with the divine. Some but not all of these inspired persons originally shared their wisdom with no intention that it serve as the impetus for forming a religion. Like any other social institution, religions are shaped not only by their founders but also by their followers and leaders (however they label their priestly class).

Religions perform what appears to be an essential service to society. Indeed, it is hard to imagine a society without some practice of honoring the spiritual element in its citizens. In our modern world, many countries, including ours, allow alternate versions of reality in multiple religions to exist side by side. At present, at least in our society, most of these alternate forms are different versions of monotheism.

We tend to think of ourselves as very enlightened because we accept this diversity without rancor for the most part. Yet, as Karen Armstrong (1993) points out, monotheism has its own weaknesses:

> Today we have become so familiar with the intolerance that has unfortunately been a characteristic of monotheism that we may not appreciate that this hostility toward other gods was a new religious attitude. Paganism was an essentially tolerant faith: provided that old cults were not threatened by the arrival of a new deity, there was always room for another god alongside the traditional pantheon. (p. 49)

We are once again in an era when that monotheistic intolerance is showing its effects worldwide: with fundamentalist groups carrying out jihads against *others,* that is, outsiders, with abortion-performing physicians being murdered, and with attacks against religious houses of worship. This is reminiscent of earlier monotheistic flaws: the Inquisition, the Crusades, even witch burning. Organized religions can be forces of good or evil.

Decisions within a religious organization may greatly distort the visions of a religion's founder or its own collected lore. For example, I think of a decision by medieval churchmen at the Council of Rome in 745 who determined that human beings were too interested in worshiping angels instead of God. In a very human decision, the Council decided to eliminate one of the four so-called Angels of Presence—dropping Uriel from the angels eligible for veneration in the church.

These very human churchmen apparently felt that they had a right to change what had previously been seen as a God-determined state in their religion. One is forced to ask how humans could simply vote to change such a divine revelation. Assuming that God created the four angels (Michael, Raphael, Gabriel, and Uriel) to fill those positions of presence (ability to stand in the presence of God), how could men assume that they could change that by a vote?

Although this particular decision was much ignored in the subsequent centuries, it illustrates the fact that religions (e.g., Judaism, Christianity, Islam, Hinduism, and Buddhism) are constantly negotiating between their founders' teachings and their human stewards' objectives in any given era. Such objectives often appear to be political (in the society or in the religious organization itself) rather than spiritual.

PRACTICALITIES IN THE NURSE'S WORLD

Why should nurses take the time to differentiate between spirituality and religion? What possible difference can that make to the nurse? These two categories comprise different domains and need to be approached differently.

We all know that when a patient has indicated his religion on a check-in form, it may or may not be meaningful. Many people who have long since quit attending any church, synagogue, temple, or mosque still list the religion of their earlier life. Many people feel that they ought to fill in this blank on the paper. Perhaps this happens in the nonchurchgoers because they still feel the same component of religion that James isolated.

On whatever basis the patient indicates (or fails to indicate) his religion, what meaning can we say that holds for the nurse? Clearly, he or she can't learn the theology of every patient, although most nurses are aware of the more unusual demands of the common religions. Yet for the nurse, the part of each religion with most importance is likely to be the component that comprises the unique personal meaning, that same slice we've already mentioned. Further, this is the same spiritual component usually held by persons without religious backgrounds. True, the nurse will on occasion encounter an atheist or agnostic who claims no relationship to a higher power. Sometimes these people hold humanistic values that provide similar, but not identical, meanings in their lives.

On the whole, it would be better if the nurse considers the spiritual aspect in every patient rather than focus on the patient's religion. Alternately, his or her theory of nursing may allow her to consider a patient's spirituality by the method of exception. That is, the nurse might consider spirituality only in those patients for whom it becomes a problem. However he or she considers the patient's spirituality, this does not permit the nurse to ignore the cultural demands of the patient's religion. These demands may be many or few and usually involve matters of ritual or life style. If the nurse does not know about these constraints, the patient or his or her family can identify them.

In Chapter 2, the nurse will find that spirituality is not an all-or-none principle. There are many levels of spirituality. People have widely different levels of sophistication and understanding when it comes to spirituality. Often such levels are revealed in the approaches people take to religion. We know, for example, that some people take religious writings as the *revealed word*, that is, something to be believed word for word. Although this approach would be measured as a low level of faith on most scales, the person at this level is likely to believe that he or she is at a high level of faith because of his or her perceived conformity with the written word.

Yet a person with a more mature faith may understand that many written words in a religion may be expressive rather than literal. Much of religion is explained in myths. The very mystery and ambiguity of such religious stories may carry significant meaning. Indeed, they usually present more depth than is recognized in the face value of such tales.

Ironically, when entering a health care system, the patient has an opportunity to list his religion but no opportunity to report his spiritual status. No health care worker asks about the patient's most important spiritual beliefs. Indeed, such a question might be difficult for a patient to answer. Identifying one's religion can usually be done with a word or two, but explaining one's spirituality might take a philosophic soliloquy of which not all are capable.

Additionally, because one's spirituality is personal rather than communal, a patient might not be inclined to share his values. In a state of health-related stress, many patients may have no desire (or capacity) to share such thoughts. True, there are patients who inspire us with their spiritual integrity, but usually this has to do with how spirituality infuses all aspects of their being rather than what they say.

Spirituality can occur outside of a religion, but the nurse may make false assumptions about the patient's spirituality (or lack of it) if he fails to identify a religious commitment. Spirituality is less visible. Often, spiritual issues reveal themselves when something in the patient's care conflicts with his value system. Issues may also arise when health issues cause a patient to reach out as he reviews his life from a spiritual perspective.

This ambiguity concerning one's spirituality is the reason behind extensive research on religion rather than on spirituality. Religion has more variables that can be correlated with health outcomes, particularly in an era like ours when nurses and others are pressed to adopt quantitative research methods. Then, as a simple example, church membership or church attendance can be easily correlated with morbidity and mortality statistics—or with other identified health care outcomes (as seen in Chapter 5).

It is easier to research variables that deal with religion rather than spirituality; religious formats or practices offer many concrete (yes/no) answers. Spirituality, on the other hand (because it means different things to different people), is harder to capture for research purposes and less amenable to quantitative measurement.

What is important to the nurse in all this complexity? First, with a few exceptions, most patients won't bring issues of spirituality or religion to the nurse's attention unless they are troubled, and almost always this disturbance will relate to the reasons for which they are in the health care system. Therefore, nurses are unlikely to be consulted for philosophic debates over spiritual matters. They are seldom asked to help the patient address complexities concerning the nature of God or other ecclesiastic matters. They are, however, often invited to explore spiritual matters when the patient or his family has lost the ability to cope with, or hope with, the existential situation.

What the patient needs from the nurse are neither intellectual answers nor blind reassurances (which are really a means of avoiding the patient's distress). What the patient most often needs is a simple human connection, to know that someone cares about him and feels his distress. Moreover, that the someone will not disappear the following day. The continuity of that caring relationship can be critical, and often that is why the nurse finds herself or himself faced with spiritual issues.

This is also why the nurse can't always pass the buck to other people (e.g., the religious professionals). The patient needs help when he or she feels the crisis. And often the best help that can be given is the very human one of the nurse being there, connecting, truly listening, and letting the patient know he is heard. This can be more important than any advice giving or any intellectual reasoning. It is also the reason why a now-and-then drop-in by a chaplain may not be felt to be as important as the ongoing relationship with the nurse.

One danger in a patient's spiritual vulnerability is that some nurses may see this as an opening to proselytize their own particular brand of religion. This, of course, is a dreadful manipulation of a patient who is vulnerable.

Much of nursing literature deals with the concepts of coping and hoping (as well as the patient's proverbial question, *why me?*). In the last analysis, what is really needed from the nurse is the human link that enables the patient to find his own coping skills, his own hopeful sentiments, and his own answers to spiritually motivated questions. Solving these spiritual challenges often gives meaning to the patient's illness, disability, or pain. Often these very challenges help a patient refocus on spiritual matters. Frequently, these existential traumas lead a patient to begin a spiritual journey. Indeed, physical or emotional distresses are often the trigger points inciting spiritual growth and development.

Why then should the nurse be able to differentiate between religion and spirituality? Simply because these elements need to be handled in different ways. The nurse can treat the religious elements of a patient's faith from a cultural or social perspective. Many of the relevant religious aspects will be codified as accepted behaviors, that is, as expected or required rituals.

However, the spiritual elements held by any patient require a different approach, a discernment by the nurse of what is important to the patient and an ability to see when the patient's values are lost or challenged in health care situations. The issue is seldom one of recognizing a spiritual problem but in knowing what, if anything, to do about it.

The best kind of help the nurse can offer is *being there,* understanding what is happening for the patient and how he feels. However, the nurse is likely to want to do something else, namely return the patient to his previous nonstressful spiritual status. To refrain from this mitigating action may require a counterintuitive stance on the part of the nurse, but that is what he or she should do.

In psychotherapy, as an analogy, there are two quite different approaches. The first one is supportive, propping up the client in his decisions, in his sense of self, and in his growing competencies. For most nurses in most caregiving situations, this sort of supportive role is almost second nature.

Yet another form of psychotherapy takes the opposite approach: taking the client deep into the morass of his feelings, leading him to understand the depths of his being. This approach aims for cure through ultimate recognition of underlying realities, but the path to getting there is not easy. Indeed, the psychotherapist must withhold false reassurances. The therapist supports the client in making the journey, but the support will be full of challenging interpretations, quite often those the patient does not want to hear. The psychotherapist must be careful not to distract the client from his or her path of exploration.

As analogy, the nurse who attempts to cut short the patient's spiritual angst is an obstruction to the patient's spiritual growth. The nurse who truly wants to work with a patient's spiritual issues must recognize that a spiritual journey assumes an uncomfortable form; the patient and his spirituality become partners and enemies struggling toward change. The patient must be allowed to toil through the spiritual trauma to the depths of understanding. His journey must not be soothed or cut short. Spiritual resolutions come with hard work. They should never be mitigated with a nurse's calming platitudes. The nurse must respect the patient's process. Nurse theorist Margaret Newman says the same thing in relation to the patient's entire being, not just his spirituality. For Newman, health is defined as expanding consciousness, and expanding consciousness is recognized in a new and higher level of organization. On the way to this new level, however, the person will have disorganized patterns. Newman (2000) describes the growth process in the following way:

> There are times when the pattern of a person becomes increasingly disorganized . . . sickness then can provide a kind of shock that reorganizes the relationships of the person's pattern in a more harmonious way (and) . . . may provide the shock that facilitates a jump from one pattern to another, presumably at a higher level of organization. (p. 12)

As to the way the nurse respects the patient's process, Newman states:

> The new paradigm of health, essential to nursing, embraces a unitary pattern of changing relationships . . . The task is not to try to change another person's pattern but to recognize it as information that depicts the whole and relate to it as it unfolds. (p. 13)

In other words, the nurse observes the patient's unfolding; he or she doesn't determine the way in which that will happen.

Yet we must acknowledge the nurse's almost instinctive desire to end the patient's struggle. This is what nurses do: They fix things. We find this same tendency echoed in many of our nursing documents. For example, the North American Nursing Diagnosis Association (NANDA, 2009) labels *spiritual distress* as a nursing diagnosis. This means that it is something to be recognized, treated, and *cured* by the nurse. He or she is to work on making it go away.

In addition, here we have the basic problem that arises in attempting to subsume spiritual goals under nursing goals. When this happens, spirituality and nursing goals are treated as if they were the *same*. The nurse will use the care patterns and behaviors he or she has learned, often without realizing that he or she has moved to a different discipline. The nurse, at least today, most often desires reaching end-state objectives with due speed. Professionals who deal with spirituality will be far more interested in the nature of the journey undertaken by the person. Indeed, slow movement may be better in many respects, giving the seeker time to integrate new understandings and new appreciations.

When the nurse chooses (or is required) to work via a predetermined set of objectives, he or she must recognize how that sets the context for care. As Newman indicates:

> . . . intervention aimed at producing a particular result becomes a problem. To intervene with a particular solution in mind is to say we know what forms the pattern of expanding consciousness will take, and we don't. (p. 97)

This is not to say that Newman's is the only theory of nursing that has a problem with preconceived outcomes. There are many. It is hoped that this illustration will serve to demonstrate that today's general preference for nursing care maps and predetermined care objectives is not without significant impact as a theoretical care model. Moreover, it has considerable (usually negative) impact on spiritually based objectives.

If the nurse using care-by-objectives theory is not spiritually mature, this may be interpreted as returning the patient to the complacency of his previous level of spiritual belief. True, a backward turning might feel more comfortable for both the patient and the nurse, but it produces a spiritual standstill. Nor is it realistic to assume that a spiritual journey can be successfully completed during the time of hospitalization—which should make spirituality a debatable nursing diagnosis, at least in this era when everything is measured in defined goals to be achieved on a timetable.

We must recognize that some phenomena (including spiritual journeys) work on a different timetable from that typically in the nurse's mind. Spiritual work is long and hard. It is not likely to end on a date specified by a bunch of normative care objectives. Nor can the nurse do the work the patient must perform for himself. One needs to ask, what is the spiritual price paid if the patient is deterred from his journey?

From a spiritual perspective, like the psychotherapist, the nurse can help by being there, actually hearing what the patient is saying, recognizing what he feels—but not by *fixing* him. Furthermore, to be there, the nurse must be present in his or her full authentic self. This form of help will assist, not obstruct, the patient in his spiritual journey. One might go so far as to break the nursing code; one might eschew empathy and allow sympathy to flow, in a human-to-human relationship.

With empathy, one puts oneself in the place of the other, seeing what that feels like. One can't really do that for the patient's spiritual journey. It doesn't work. If the nurse attempts to see how it feels, he or she will only see how it would feel for the nurse, not how it feels for the patient.

SUMMARY

Why then must the nurse differentiate between spirituality and religion? The answer is simple: They require very different nursing approaches. A patient's religion is a communal relationship. It can be addressed as a cultural phenomenon. It can be handled with respect and support by asking the patient and/or family about the religious constraints and by respecting the patient's right to his own beliefs.

If, on the other hand, the patient's health care situation had led him into the sort of spiritual distress that initiates a true seeking of new spiritual meanings, then the nurse must restrain from the urge to make things comfortable, to subvert that difficult journey. The nurse must learn to tolerate the patient's spiritual pain along his path.

Much of nursing has to do with hiding from the patient. *Professionalism* becomes a mask: "Of course, I don't mind that you're naked—I'm a nurse." Even the uniform is a psychological barrier. It requires great courage on the nurse's part to drop that distancing self-protection so as to really help a patient on a spiritual journey. The words that Nouwen (1972) offers to seminarians could also apply to nurses. He says:

> . . . no one can help anyone without becoming involved, without entering with his whole person into the painful situation, without taking the risk of becoming hurt, wounded or even destroyed in the process. (p. 72)

Nurses are not used to this kind of advice, but if a nurse wants to accompany a patient on a spiritual journey, the nurse's responses will call for this same level of commitment. Are nurses prepared for helping, not hindering, patients on spiritual journeys? Indeed, not every nurse will be able to achieve the mind-set this transition demands.

REFERENCES

Armstrong, K. (1993). *A history of God: The 4,000-year quest of Judaism, Christianity and Islam.* New York: Ballantine Books.

James, W. (1997). *The varieties of religious experience.* New York: Simon & Schuster (A Touchstone Book).

Newman, M. A. (2000). *Health as expanding consciousness* (2nd ed.). Sudbury, MA: Jones and Bartlett Publishers.

Nouwen, H. J. M. (1972). *The wounded healer.* New York: Doubleday, Image Books.

BIBLIOGRAPHY

North American Nursing Diagnosis Association. (2009). In T. H. Herdman (Ed.), *Nursing diagnoses: Definitions and classification, 2009–2011.* Hoboken, NJ: Wiley & Blackwell.

CHAPTER 2

Levels of Spiritual Development: What Happens When the Nurse and the Patient Differ?

As many researchers assert, are there really levels of spiritual development? If so, our systems of care make no adjustments when nurses and patients are on different levels. Indeed, to do so would be highly unrealistic. Testing for levels of spiritual development, as we will see, is a complex thing under any researched classification, and not all patients would be in a mindset or physical state where such testing would be possible. For example, a person recently affected by stroke might not have the verbal skills required.

Moreover, in all systems of spiritual classification, it is impossible for people at a lower level to truly understand the thoughts and feelings of people at higher levels. Yet these differences in levels may be the source of many spiritual issues between nurse and patient. How do we resolve such issues when they arise?

We have all seen instances when nurses and patients fail to connect over spiritual matters. Sometimes it's as simple as a patient asking, "Why did God do this to me?" And the nurse offering an answer that avoids the question, such as, "I'm sure you're going to be fine." Or a nurse saying, "I'll pray for you," and a patient responding, "I don't believe in that stuff."

This chapter suggests that the reason such clashes occur often is because the patient and the nurse are at different levels of spiritual development. Obviously, other factors could be at fault, but in this chapter, we'll examine the problems caused by different levels.

What *does* happen when the nurse and the patient are at different levels of spiritual development? To answer this question, we must first look at spiritual development through two different lenses. Initially, we must ask, is spirituality a natural stage of growth and development in human beings? Then we must ask, within spiritual development, are there deepening stages of spiritual maturity? Once we have answered these questions, we'll be ready to get back to our practical nursing question concerning what happens when the nurse and the patient differ in levels of spirituality.

IS SPIRITUAL GROWTH A NATURAL STAGE OF DEVELOPMENT IN HUMAN BEINGS?

Respected psychologists and philosophers have posed many models of growth and development for both individuals and groups of people. Some of these models incorporate spiritual elements, some don't. Earlier models tended to avoid spiritual elements, probably because of the complexities involved. A few illustrations of both types of models are discussed.

PSYCHOLOGICAL MODELS FOR THE INDIVIDUAL

Most nurses are already familiar with various psychological schemes describing human growth and development. Certainly, they are familiar with the classic works of Jean Piaget, Erik Erikson, and Abraham Maslow. Piaget (1976) particularly investigated early childhood learning, so we won't examine his work here because the child has little concept of spirituality.

Erikson (1985), on the other hand, goes farther, proposing a series of developmental life tasks, each of which needs to be achieved before the next higher task can be tackled. These tasks have become classic in developmental theory, and nurses will recall them. When successfully achieved, the infant develops basic trust rather than mistrust. The child completes three tasks: developing autonomy versus shame and doubt, initiative versus guilt, and industry versus inferiority. The adolescent acquires identity versus role confusion, and the young adult strives for intimacy versus isolation. The adult task of generativity versus stagnation follows, with the rest of life devoted to the single task of establishing ego integrity versus despair. It's difficult to read spirituality into Erikson's *ego integrity*, although for some individuals that might be a part of spirituality. But, on the whole, Erikson doesn't address our subject matter of spirituality.

Abraham Maslow (1970) was one of the pioneers to move beyond the traditional psychological phases. His original developmental phases were physiological needs, safety needs, needs for love and belonging, esteem needs, the need for self-actualization, the need to know and understand, and aesthetic needs. His stages were messier than Erikson's in that they were only more or less serial, and might be altered in sequence for some people. There was a path, but it wasn't rigid and lock-step.

More interestingly, Maslow's (1971) later research, dealt with a phenomenon that escaped his earlier classification system and bordered on the spiritual. He investigated what he termed *Being-values* (peak experiences). Being-values included such things as moments of rapture and transcendence. Some people might interpret such peak experiences as spiritual; others might avoid that classification.

Nevertheless, many people have such peak experiences in association with spiritual moments. I recall, for example, a patient describing just such a moment when he or she sat in the hospital chapel, and experienced the sun coming through a stained glass window, falling on him as if he or she were its target.

It would be inaccurate to pose Being-values as constituting a separate life phase for Maslow; he saw these experiences as unique and momentary incidents. They did not constitute a stable and sustained way of being in the world. Yet he did speak of two classes of people: those who were *merely* self-actualized and the self-actualized peakers. Maslow's Being-values involved things directly perceived, not learned. And the incidences in which these peak experiences occurred had what many would call spiritual qualities.

Theorists who came later moved to stages of human development beyond the familiar phases proposed by early-stage theorists. Ken Wilber (1986) outstripped the more traditional Western developmental models put forth by Erikson and Maslow and introduced life phases that explicitly moved into spiritual realms.

His early transpersonal developmental model added Eastern models virtually atop of Western models—as if the latter had simply stopped too soon. Wilber proposed 10 phases of human development, with early stages resembling those of Piaget and other developmental psychologists, but the final added phases lead to various spiritual states. For example, of his Stage Seven, *psychic opening*, he says ". . . the individual's cognitive and perceptual capacities apparently become so pluralistic and universal that they begin to 'reach beyond' any narrowly personal or individual perspectives and concerns" (p. 72).

And he claims that *subtle* Stage Eight is the seat of archetypes and of transcendent insight, clearly a step further along a spiritual path than Stage Seven.

Causal Stage Nine is where he says the usual ego is subordinated and: ". . . a wide cosmic perception and feeling of boundless universal self replaces it . . . a being which is in essence one with the Supreme Self" (pp. 49–50).

Wilber's *Ultimate* Stage Ten is where consciousness awakens to its eternal abode as absolute Spirit. Clearly, all of Wilber's final stages deal with experiential, not intellectual, spiritual changes. These are experiences that literally change the person.

Later, Wilber moved from transpersonal psychology to what he called an integral philosophy or psychology in which he further developed and integrated developmental spiritual systems. Two of Wilber's books (2000 and 2007) deal specifically with spirituality from that expanded perspective.

Stanislav Grof (1988) proposed a simpler developmental scheme, contrasting *hylotropic* consciousness (matter oriented, i.e., everyday) with *holotropic* consciousness (aiming toward the whole and characterized by nonordinary psychological states, i.e., meditative, mystical, or psychedelic). Like Wilber, his holotropic consciousness has differentiated subtle and causal realms.

Wilber and Grof present developmental schemas in which advanced levels of spirituality are natural phases of human growth and development. Most Eastern models of development, in contrast to Western ones, include stages of development we would label as spiritual. The reader who wishes to explore such models might start with Aurobindo (McDermott, 1987).

DEVELOPMENTAL MODELS FOR COMMUNITIES AND ORGANIZATIONS

Developmental models may be extended beyond the individual, to groups and organizations. A good example is the Spiral Dynamics model because, unlike many others, its higher stages include moral and spiritual values.

Following the original work of Clare Graves, Don Beck and Christopher Cowan (1996) identify orienting worldviews that evolve in a developmental spiral. They apply these worldviews to many organizational and institutional domains in addition to individual human development.

Beck and Cowan give a sort of psychocultural DNA that structures the mind-set of an individual or an organization, with implications for deepening spiritual values at different Meme levels. *Memes*, as they call them, are collections of compatible philosophic elements, including a worldview, a valuing system, a description of psychological reality, and a way of thinking that seems natural to those living within a given Meme. Each Meme system represents a different way of seeing the world. Indeed, one must step outside of a Meme to even recognize its existence.

Beck and Cowan arrange these Memes in a hierarchy, where higher Memes show a more developed sense of ethics and morality. These different

Memes are reflected in the traits of organizations that come into being under different circumstances. As we briefly describe these Memes, the reader might want to envision how a patient care unit is managed or even the way a health care institution is organized and run.

Beck and Cowan identify their Memes by a color scheme for simplicity. Because each Meme stands for a collection of variables, this is a good tool for the reader. Only a few simple indicators will be given here for each Meme, and one needs to understand that each Meme is actually a much more complex system. The reader will benefit by checking out the full details that are presented in Beck and Cowan's book. Each Meme could be a book in itself because it contains all elements of a philosophy, a set of values, ways of relating to others and to power structures, ways of thinking, and ways of viewing reality. Each Meme has a large group of compatible elements that make up a total life style of the complex community that employs it.

Beginning at the bottom of the scale, the *Beige Meme* has a philosophy motivated by the primitive desire to stay alive. At this level, loose bands of people form for the purpose of survival. Organization is simple and stark: People do what it takes to stay alive. Seldom does the Beige Meme matter to us in health care organizations, but one might envision some battlefield conditions which come close.

In a less technological age, I can recall being taught a course called *Battlefield Nursing*. The first directive in that course was to first treat those more likely to survive. The more compromised victims were taken care of later—if there was time. Potential for survival was the criterion applied in such battlefield situations then. It's possible that today some EMT crews may run into similar situations.

Beck and Cowan's *Purple Meme* rises above mere survival but is still too primitive to give much attention to mature spiritual values, although it includes magic, ritual, and blood relationships. Magic and ritual in early societies might indeed be part of the spiritual values of the time. This romanticized era might take us back to thinking of health care in the era of the Druids: herbs and visions. Perhaps some early Knight Templars' hospitals came close as well, as they had little to offer in the way of medical care beyond comfort at the time of death. Spirituality was probably their main therapy, although the delivery was in the form of religious ritual.

The next level, the *Red Meme*, deals mostly with power and aggressiveness, and it also is deficient in spiritual values. Might makes right here. The leader controls the rewards and punishments of others. He provides security, even though his methods are exploitive.

The *Blue Meme* gives us a beginning focus on some values that may relate to spirituality: service, loyalty, and obedience to the rules. The environment has become less threatening. Partly that's because the *right* answers have been found—and are to be followed. Regulations and a code of conduct set the pattern that all are expected to follow. There is less exploitation but no room for individuality or deviance from the plan. The process is authoritarian and hierarchical and thinking is absolutistic. For example, a nurse wouldn't think of questioning a physician's order.

In nursing, some of these Blue Meme situations occurred in hospitals under various religious orders. Often the given religion was incorporated into the lives of the Meme's members. In this era, many nurses were required to begin their work days with compulsory religious services.

I recall meeting many older nurses who had entered nursing under a Blue Meme system. They had been made to choose between a married life and a life dedicated to nursing. They were not given the option of having both. When I first started working as a young nurse, some of them had a wonderful dedication to nursing, as if it were a spiritual calling. Others resented the fact that the younger nurses were allowed to have a fuller life than had been offered to them. But right or wrong, religion-bound rules fit comfortably into the Blue Meme ideology.

The next situation, the *Orange Meme*, deals primarily with competition and winning, still a long way from spirituality as a motivator. Under an Orange Meme, autonomous behavior has slipped into a changed worldview. Focus in the Orange Meme is on success and self-reliance. The competitive manipulator is the winner here. Not surprisingly, this model dominated just when nursing decided to make itself a professional career, competing to join the academic world. Often this move was achieved by setting up nursing against medicine, with nursing having its own values, its own research, and its own domain. One might contrast this Meme with the then Russian system in which nursing was a step in the ladder toward becoming a physician. One will recognize the Orange Meme still in existence in some health care organizations. Indeed, one can find examples of the Blue Meme as well.

Beck and Cowan's *Green Meme* is the first shift that reflects values that might be spiritual in a modern sense. In this complex, one cares about the well-being of the group members and the building of consensus among them. Cooperation replaces competition here. Caring and reconciliation matter. One might imagine concepts such as team nursing coming into being under the Green Meme. That system, of course, looked to build teams rather than hierarchies. Additionally, the focus shifted from an orientation on tasks to the people-oriented focus on patients. And a people-oriented focus opens the possibility of spiritual values.

The next two Memes are the forms toward which many of our health care organizations are now growing, and they are even more directly connected to spiritual values. At least Beck and Cowan mark these as making a qualitative shift in that direction.

The *Yellow Meme* is flexible and knowledge based. In nursing, we see trends such as valuing competency more than rank. Nursing specialists and nurse practitioners come on the scene under this Meme. Outcome-based management allows for experimentation with different work plans. Effort is taken to use people for their talents. Experiments may allow different forms of organization: different work hours, different plans for different employees. The individual becomes important in a caring way rather than just being seen as a tool of management.

Spiritual elements include Beck and Cowan's statements such as:

> The interactive universe is becoming more intriguing than autonomy or even community. (p. 275)

> Values come from the magnificence of existence rather than selfish or group interest. They are inherent within the nature of life itself—fundamental, natural laws. (p. 279)

The *Turquoise Meme* takes the next developmental step with a holistic focus and a recognized desire to bring together mind and spirit. Here the authors say:

> Self is part of larger, conscious, spiritual whole that also serves itself. (p. 287)

> At TURQUOISE, one stands in awe of the cosmic order, the creative forces that exist from the Big Bang to the smallest molecule. (p. 291)

As one can see that these Meme structures grow and change as situations evolve. In any organization, one can probably find a mixture of Memes, with change taking place toward a higher level of development.

Although we're not ready yet to ask about how the level of spiritual development affects nursing, we can't help but recognize that mixes and mismatches of Meme levels could take place. Suppose, for example, an ambitious new nursing vice president comes into a position determined to improve the quality of nursing, her head full of all the wonderful Yellow Meme principles she has learned in her schooling. Then let's assume that she fails to recognize that she is bringing all these ideals into an institution that is still primarily in the Orange Meme phase.

To assume that people can jump from Orange to Yellow without any intermediate steps is like assuming a child can go directly from addition and subtraction to calculus. Imagine that people who have always acted competitively against each other are expected to work together cooperatively and be sensitive to each others' needs. Indeed, I think this is why so many consultants who come into an institution with a readymade *solution* in their back pocket fail. One cannot bring about change while failing to notice where one is beginning. Assessing the operating Meme of an organization is where one starts. Today we can still find health care organizations in all colors, so to speak.

Given the above models for individual and group spiritual maturity, it seems that we have a positive answer to our first question: Is spirituality a natural stage of growth and development in human beings? Growth toward spiritual goals may not be inevitable, but it certainly is possible. The models given here are representative of the many developmental models that may be found. And these examples should be adequate to make the point that at least some theorists see aspects of spirituality emerging as developmental stages, both in individuals and in groups. Hence, we are ready to move on to our second question: Are there deepening stages of spirituality?

ARE THERE STAGES OF SPIRITUAL GROWTH?

To answer the second question, we must look to developmental schemas that deal more directly with spirituality. We'll look at two examples here: those of James Fowler and of M. Scott Peck. Both these authors assert that spirituality in the individual can develop and grow.

Fowler's (1981) developmental schema is perhaps the best researched system, and his book, *Stages of Faith*, has become the classic for differentiating among stages of spiritual growth. His stages are not unlike the stages of other developmental theorists in that they tend to correspond loosely with age. Fowler is careful to explain that his notion of faith is not synonymous with religion, although religion may mark the way in which spirituality is expressed by many people. Faith, for Fowler, rests in beliefs concerning ultimate meaningful values in a person's life.

Like Cowan and Beck's developmental model, there are many variables in Fowler's system and the few elements that will be given here are merely illustrative, not meant to make the reader capable of applying the system. Indeed, Fowler's interviewers required careful training to assess subjects. You could say that Fowler created sets of spiritual Memes.

Despite the oversimplification here, we will loosely differentiate Fowler's six stages of faith. The early stages are more closely tied to the child's general developmental abilities than the later stages. Stage One, occurring when the child is perhaps 3–7 years of age, is fantasy-filled and is imitative. Fowler labels this as *intuitive-projective faith*. This stage is marked by fantasy unrestrained by logic and may therefore contain both good and destructive images. Essentially, it follows other developmental theorists' explanations of the child's thought patterns at this age.

Fowler's Stage Two, *mythic-literal faith*, is similarly attached to developmental psychology in that it rests in stories and beliefs of the child's community. This phase is typical of the school child, unreflective and given to literal interpretations.

Stage Three, *synthetic-conventional faith*, begins in adolescence. It is marked by yielding authority to forces external to the self, and rests primarily in the person's interpersonal sensitivity. It is seen as an extension of what is experienced with other people. The viewpoint is conformist and tuned to the expectations of significant others.

Yet the beliefs and values are deeply felt at this stage, although they haven't been evaluated. This is logical because most persons at this stage of faith are not yet sure of their own identities. Hence, placing spirituality in a force beyond themselves makes sense. Ironically, people at this stage may appear more religious and more spiritual than people who may actually be at higher stages of faith. Stage Three faith, because it rests in forces external to the person, is often associated with religious communities.

In one era, let's say the late 40s and early 50s, when most nursing students came directly from high school graduation, this stage probably marked most of our entering students. One can see that becoming nuns marked a different enactment of the same sense of spirituality, especially by women of this young age.

It is interesting to think of the disjunction created for such young women in the late 50s and early 60s when nursing leaders began to shift the ideology of nursing toward the scientific and academic. Imagine this group (young women were still the typical students then), drawn into nursing by a notion of spiritual devotion to mankind in keeping with their Stage Three level of faith. Then picture them finding themselves instead, inculcated into an ideology that valued scientific dispassion instead of spiritual values.

Fowler's Stage Three probably marks the first spiritual stage where many people remain fixated, dropping off the spiritual growth curve. Indeed, we all know people, young and old, who remain in Stage Three, taking comfort in its reliance on a power outside of themselves.

Fowler's Stage Four, *individuative-reflective faith*, represents a major shift in the spiritual progression. This stage normally occurs in late adolescence or young adulthood. Here the person begins to take serious responsibility for his or her own commitments, including commitment to a given faith structure.

This is where true individuality versus being defined by group membership, rears its head. As I write this, I keep thinking of that old classic film, *Rebel Without a Cause*. Indeed that's how many young people at this phase appear. They are in rebellion against all the things that identified them merely as members of given groups.

In terms of faith, this is when they struggle to give old religious symbols intellectual meaning, and they struggle to find themselves as separate persons. It is not surprising that in struggling with conventional systems supporting spiritual values (usually religious affiliations), rebellion may be the most commonly exhibited behavior by many. Although this stage may begin in rebellion, many people find reconciliation, which may involve leaving past beliefs behind or reinterpreting past beliefs in larger or different contexts. Yet rebellion stands out as a major characteristic of Stage Four.

Ironically, this forecasts a major problem in which a religious young nurse deals with a patient who appears to have rejected all thought of spirituality in his rebellion phase. Where the nurse is seeing such spiritual struggles as negative on the part of a patient, the situation may cast the nurse in the role of obstructing the patient's spiritual maturing. It is easier for the spiritually immature nurse to suggest that the patient return to prior beliefs than to support his struggle for a new definition of spirituality—especially if she has yet to reach her own struggle between Stages Three and Four.

Yet ironically, the patient is actually ahead of the very religious nurse in his spiritual advancement. Recall here that, although the beginning of these stages of faith tends to be associated with age, we actually find people of all ages at each stage of faith.

This may be the first place where we get a glimmer of a problem discussed in Chapter 4: whether spiritual goals or healing goals take precedence. Should spiritual work only be encouraged if it supports healing? Or is that putting a more important value into the service of a lesser value? When one is in the health field, health goals have a tendency to be given priority over spiritual goals.

Differences in levels of spiritual maturity may also inhibit conversations between nurse and patient, no matter what direction the inequality takes. In other words, in assuming spiritual care as part of their obligation, nurses may be taking on an assignment for which they are ill prepared in their own development as well as in their knowledge.

One can understand why nursing curricula don't usually deal with spirituality, except perhaps to present the student with a few religious conventions. Often these conventions deal with food selection and preparation, prayer requirements, and clothing. When spiritual values include refusing modern medical therapy, however, especially for dependent children, courts have frequently imposed modern medicine over parents' stated beliefs.

Fowler's next stage is called *conjunctive faith* (Stage Five). Stage Five has a tolerance for diversity that neither Stage Three nor Stage Four could endure. At this stage, as Fowler describes it, the person has a sense of detachment that allows him to let the world reveal itself as it is. Stage Five can probably be best illustrated in a quote from Fowler's work:

> Whereas Stage Four could afford to equate self pretty much with its own conscious awareness of self, Stage Five must come to terms with its own unconscious—the unconscious personal, social and species or archetypal elements that are partly determinative of our actions and responses. (p. 186)

Not surprisingly, this is a level of faith that not everyone achieves.

Stage Six, Fowler's last stage, is called *universalizing faith*. It is transcendent and rarely achieved. At this stage, people sense an ultimate environment that is inclusive of all being as Fowler describes it. This is the culmination phase of faith that few reach. Fowler gives examples such as Gandhi and Mother Teresa.

M. Scott Peck's (1993) description of spiritual stages is simpler than Fowler's, yet traces, as he admits, very similar patterns. Peck has fewer stages and associates them perhaps more closely to religion. His Stage One is labeled *chaotic/antisocial*. The person at Peck's Stage One is unprincipled and antisocial; he or she is self-serving and manipulative. One might call this a negative spiritual stage.

Peck's Stage Two is called *formal/institutional*, and is very dependent on some institution. Although a church is the main source, he also mentions structuring institutions such as prisons and the military. One can see many comparisons to Fowlers Stage Three, but Peck adds an interesting analysis of why churchgoers have such an attachment to the institutional rituals. Perceived threats to these organizing rituals (e.g., when churches attempt to change aspects of their liturgies) can be very threatening to members. As Peck succinctly states of people at this stage:

> . . . their vision of God is almost entirely that of an external being. They have very little understanding of that half of God which lives inside each of us. . . . (p. 123)

Peck calls his Stage Three *skeptic/individual*, and it closely resembles Fowler's Stage Four, albeit with a bit more focus on the overt rebellion aspects. He says that the people in this stage are not religious in the ordinary sense but are not antisocial either.

Peck's final Stage Four is labeled *mystical/communal*, and includes people who can see, as he says, "a cohesion beneath the surface of things" (p. 125). They not only tolerate ambiguity but are also comfortable with it. Peck notes that this stage of mystery occurs in virtually all religions, including Christianity, Islam, Taoism, Buddhism, and Hinduism.

Although both Fowler and Peck give us developmental stages of spirituality, it is frustrating that the similar stages are differently numbered. But, in any case, we have two examples here of spirituality occurring with its own developmental stages.

But not everyone who examines spirituality is a developmentalist. For example, William Bloom (1994) identifies the following forms as simply three basic styles of spirituality rather than levels. He illustrates *mystical abandon* by dance, *devotional aspiration* by prayer, and *contemplation* as dominated by thought.

In any case, we have now identified systems of individual growth and development that include spiritual levels and models of spirituality that are based on levels. Hence, we are ready to come back to our original question: What happens when the nurse and the patient are at different levels of spiritual development?

WHAT HAPPENS WHEN THE NURSE AND THE PATIENT ARE AT DIFFERENT LEVELS OF SPIRITUAL DEVELOPMENT?

Perhaps the first thing of importance in looking at different spiritual levels of maturity between nurse and patient is the fact that, even if one has intellectual knowledge of higher states than one's own, that knowledge doesn't have an experiential impact. The person is more likely to act on where he or she is than on what information he or she has received in a class.

Immediately, we understand that spirituality is one of those subjects that is internalized by experience and/or inculcation. For example, a Blue Meme experience where the environment involved a total life dedicated to nursing was more likely to inculcate a level of spirituality than a modern nursing class giving students an intellectual understanding of diverse religious practices.

I'll illustrate this discussion, with Fowler's stage numbers because they've been more thoroughly researched than Peck's, although the discussion would be similar in any case. Many people at Fowler's higher stages of spiritual maturity, let's say Stages Five or Six, would have tolerance for those at lower stages. A patient at these stages, for example, might have great insight into a nurse at Stage Three. Ordinarily, he or she would have no need to confront or try to change her.

On the other hand, I've seen a patient probably at Stage Five faith demand that an avid Stage Three nurse leave his room. He was in severe pain at the time and simply didn't have the patience for her well-intended Stage Three proselytizing. It was a case where they both knew that he was dying. He was comfortable with that knowledge, whereas she was afraid that he would die without the blessings of her church.

Such direct proselytizing is seldom a problem today. Nurses are taught to respect every patient's religious beliefs, and, for the most part, they follow that directive. With the present growth toward a global community, today's nurse is exposed to people from many different faiths, with many different beliefs.

Yet lack of understanding spiritual *levels* can become a problem. As I indicated in Chapter 1, we even see this problem in our nursing documents. The example I gave there was the nursing diagnosis of *spiritual distress* as labeled by the North American Nursing Diagnosis Association (2009). Classification as a diagnosis means that the item is something to be recognized and treated by the nurse. Returning the patient to his original level of spirituality (that might be Fowler's Level Three) would probably be labeled as a good solution in this case. The patient's struggle or rebellion at the beginning of Stage Four would be seen as something to be eschewed.

Indeed, the clash between Fowler's Stages Three and Four may be responsible for the most common spiritual problems seen in nursing practice. It would be an interesting study for someone to read the contemporary nursing literature regarding spirituality in terms of its level of spiritual development. My suspicion from my own casual reading is that most of the nursing literature would conform to Stage Three values.

Furthermore, adjusting to a new stage of spiritual development is seldom easy for the individual, and the possibility of advancement may be brought on by something catastrophic like a serious illness. Unfortunately, the nurse's playbook almost invariably suggests that ferment in a patient be calmed down, not enhanced or even let alone.

Alternately, the nurse also is exposed to tragic and stressful situations in the health care environment. And it may be the nurse who is struggling in reaching a new level of spirituality. A nurse at Stage Four may have difficulty dealing with a patient at Stage Three. The smug certainty of the patient may threaten the nurse's spiritual journey. Nurses also fall prey to depression if they work in a particularly difficult area of practice, and this may enhance the likelihood of their own spiritual maturing. Spiritual advancement, alas, is often hard work and mind absorbing at best.

If spirituality is more a matter of maturing or inculcation rather than learning, then nurses, physicians, and other health care workers may be out of their depth. Unfortunately, as relates to high-level patients, the same may be true of some hospital chaplains.

Yet existentially it is quite true that nurses are faced with spirituality-related questions by patients in situations where not to answer would be difficult. Conditions surrounding death and permanent injury often bring up religious or spiritual questions. Perhaps the most common question from patients (as mentioned earlier) is some form of the question, "Why did God do this to me?" This is usually a Stage Three or Four question, and the patient is seldom seeking the philosophical analysis such a question would actually invoke. The nurse may best understand that a response of touch or of simply *Being There* (see Dossey, Keegan, & Guzzetta, 2000) may be an adequate response.

Requests by the patient or family for spirituality *therapy* from the nurse may involve a request for prayers of an intercessionary nature. Suppose, for example, that the nurse is asked to pray for the survival of a patient who is critical. Here the nurse has the right to respond based on her own spiritual beliefs. Yet a negative response on her part may be a source of alienating a patient or his family.

The nurse must be sensitive enough to know answering such questions or requests with sensitivity may be more important than the content of the specific answer. Just knowing that there are spiritual levels, may help the nurse deal with such matters. We would hope that every nurse has a spiritual sensitivity that at the very least makes him or her consider the patient's spiritual quandaries as worthy of concern. Simply conveying that recognition may be the most important nursing act. There are no perfect answers to any of these nurse/patient situations. As in so many cases, it all depends on the particular relationship between the patient and the nurse.

Near-death experiences (NDEs) on the part of a patient may also bring up spiritual questions (see Chapter 3). These experiences are usually felt by the patient to come from a very high level (usually a new level) of spirituality. In these cases, the nurse will do well to respect the patient's encounter and not try to negate its reality for the patient. Indeed, it may help the patient to know that many others have had similar experiences when pronounced dead.

It is not really up to the staff to interpret what that experience means to the patient. But they do need to know that an NDE may be a very important experience for the patient. So many health care workers feel a necessity to rush in and reassure the patient that the encounter was simply a matter of the brain lacking oxygen, that is, just an hallucination. This need to bring about a premature closure seems to serve the worker far more than the patient.

It's not possible to elaborate all the situations that may occur relative to differences in spiritual levels between nurse and patient. We are simply trying to illustrate the problems that can arise when such differences occur. Challenges and failures occur when a nurse chooses (or is forced) to take on a subject for which he or she is ill equipped. Unfortunately, some nurses who are well indoctrinated in their own religion may assume they have more knowledge in this area than they do.

Some subject matters may be taught—they deal mostly with content and processes. Other subjects must be internalized through processes of inculcation. For example, a nurse may admire and attempt to internalize the ability of a mentor to handle spiritual situations. In other cases, spiritual maturity and the ability to handle spiritual conflicts with patients may depend on the nurse's growth in her own life. Knowledge and the ability for action in such cases is one of the greatest challenges for nursing because it cannot be planned, taught, or subjected to a list of objectives.

SUMMARY

To deal effectively with patients' states of spirituality requires a great deal of knowledge about a subject matter (spirituality) that is really its own domain. Successfully handling spiritual issues requires a level of personal spiritual maturity on the part of the nurse. Yet we make no spiritual requirements of nurses in their education or in their qualifications for hire. Nurses have different levels of spirituality and knowledge in this domain.

We don't live in an era when spiritual values can be forcibly inculcated in a nursing population (fortunately). Yet where spiritually mature nurses exhibit sensitivity to patients' needs, other nurses may benefit from modeling the behaviors of the mature nurses.

Still in many cases, nurses include aspects of spirituality as part of their normal work. Indeed, spiritual issues may be imposed on them by the situations that emerge. Spirituality cannot be reduced to a procedure, although nurses can grow in their knowledge of it by carefully designed educational programs and, even more, by life experiences.

It is difficult but not impossible to respect the clashes of philosophies out of which both nurses and patients draw their spiritual values. In most cases, nursing care doesn't demand that these differences be specifically addressed. A sensitive humanistic approach is often the best approach for the nurse.

To return to our original question, it does appear that spiritual levels exist. Various researchers have made similar descriptions of these levels. And it appears that some of the early levels of development are more characterized by a naïve certainty than is true of more developed levels. This leaves the path open for nurses at lower levels to attempt to manipulate spiritual responses of patients. Some patients actually may already be at higher states than the nurses who are filled with certainties about what is best. When nurses deal with spiritual matters, it is clear that this mind-set leaves open the possibility for collision between patient and nurse.

REFERENCES

Beck, D. E., & Cowan, C. C. (1996). *Spiral dynamics: Mastering values, leadership, and change.* Oxford, UK: Blackwell Publishing.

Fowler, James W. (1981). *Stages of faith: The psychology of human development and the quest for meaning.* San Francisco: HarperSanFrancisco.

Peck, M. S. (1993). *Further along the road less traveled: The unending journey toward spiritual growth.* New York: Simon & Schuster.

Wilber, K. (1986). The spectrum of development. In K. Wilber, J. Engler, & D. P. Brown (Eds.), *Transformations of consciousness: Conventional and contemplative perspectives on development* (pp. 65–105). Boston: Random House.

BIBLIOGRAPHY

Bloom, W. (1994). First steps: An introduction to spiritual practice. In A. Walker (Ed.), *The kingdom within: A guide to the spiritual work of the Findhorn Community* (pp. 158–165). Moray, Scotland: Findhorn Press.

Dossey, B. M., Keegan, L., & Guzzetta, C. E. (2000). *Holistic nursing: A handbook for practice* (3rd ed.). Gaithersburg, MD: Aspen Publishers.

Erikson, E. H. (1985). *Childhood and society* (2nd ed.). New York: W.W. Norton & Company.

Erikson, E. H., Erikson, J. M., & Kivnick, H. (1986). *Vital involvement in old age.* New York: W.W. Norton & Company.

Grof, S. (1988). *The adventure of self-discovery.* Albany, NY: The State University of New York Press.

Maslow, A. H. (1970). *Motivation and personality* (2nd ed.). New York: Harper and Row.

Maslow, A. H. (1971). *The farther reaches of human nature* (2nd ed.). New York: Viking Press.

McDermott, R. (Ed.). (1987). *The essential Aurobindo.* Hudson, NY: Lindisfarne Press.

North American Nursing Diagnosis Association. (2009). In T. H. Herdman (Ed.), *Nursing diagnoses: Definitions and classification, 2009–2011.* Hoboken, NJ: Wiley & Blackwell.

Piaget, J. (1976). The stages of intellectual development in childhood and adolescence. In H. E. Gruber & J. J. Voneche (Eds.), *The essential Piaget* (pp. 814–819). New York: Basic Books.

Wilber, K. (2000). *Sex, ecology, spirituality: The spirit of evolution* (2nd ed., rev.). Boston: Shambhala.

Wilber, K. (2007). *Integral spirituality: A startling new role for religion in the modern and postmodern world.* Boston: Integral Books.

CHAPTER 3

Spirituality and the Brain:
Is Spirituality Programmed
in the Brain?

In medicine and in the minds of many nurses, there is a notion that, if it's in the brain then it can't have any external reality. For example, just this week yet another physician boldly announced in an Internet piece that near-death experiences (NDEs) have no validity and that they are strictly traceable to events in the brain. This pronouncement clearly caused distress and confusion in a woman who, in the same piece, was describing her own very meaningful NDE. There tends to be a great challenge, particularly to any spiritual phenomena, in the medical ideology.

Each nurse needs to examine her own thoughts and feelings on this issue: Can a thing be in the brain and still have a spiritual reality? Is this disjuncture between brain events and spiritual events to be accepted without questioning? Or are there vulnerabilities in this position? Before the nurse makes a judgment on this issue, it is important to know how far medical research has come in tracking spiritual events and their correlations with brain events. This chapter will address those advances.

We tend to think of spirituality as a mind-set acquired through certain life experiences. Indeed, we often think that nurses may be more spiritual than most people. We make that assumption because they have entered a helping profession, one with perhaps fewer fiscal rewards, inconvenient hours, and serious job performance pressures. Yet in truth, we also have nurses who

---

Some materials in this chapter have been adapted from content in Barnum, B., *Mystic Encounters: The Door Ajar*.

enter the profession entirely for other reasons, for example, job security in an insecure world.

Spiritual values may emerge from life experiences, but there are also ways in which the brain fosters such values. We might, for example, look at the temporal-limbic system to find our first illustration of programming for spiritual experiences.

THE TEMPORAL-LIMBIC SYSTEM

The temporal lobes are immediately beneath the ears on both sides of the head. Adjacent to the temporal lobe are underlying structures of the *limbic system*. The limbic system is on the medial (inner) surface of the cerebral hemisphere, surrounding the upper part of the brainstem, nested beneath the corpus callosum, which connects the right and left sides of the brain. The limbic system is sometimes called the mammalian brain, and it is thought to have emerged in human evolution before the cerebral cortex. This part of the brain is unconscious but has profound effects on the conscious cortex. It is known to generate certain emotions, appetites, and behavioral urges related to survival. Yet some of those emotions, the spiritual ones, might be seen as going far beyond survival tactics.

The temporal lobe-limbic system is thought to be responsible for many of the most spiritually transcendent experiences known to human beings. Typically, these events are traced to nerve excitation in the right temporal lobe. Rita Carter (1998) describes these spiritual experiences as occurring in:

> . . . an area in the temporal lobe of the brain that appears to produce intense feelings of spiritual transcendence, combined with a sense of some mystical presence. (p. 13)

She notes that, when stimulated, this area produces such feelings even in nonreligious people. She reports people seeing a presence and a light. When this experience can be measured, an electroencephalogram (EEG) shows a spike and slow-wave seizure over the temporal lobe.

Temporal-limbic events include the NDE, and that may be the spiritual encounter that most often falls under the medical lens. NDEs will be the next physiological event discussed in this chapter. But for the moment, let's stay with other spiritual effects from the temporal-limbic system. It is important to keep in mind that these are physiological events separate from the belief system of the person experiencing an NDE.

Usually as nurses, we are dealing with patients who have irregularities in the following components of the limbic system:

1. *Hypothalamus*—creates numerous subtle adjustments, adapting the body to its environment, regulating body temperature, genital function, sleep, food intake (subtle adjustments), permits long-term memory.
2. *Hippocampus*—encoding station, lays down conscious memory.
3. *Thalamus*—major sensory relay station, directs incoming information to various parts of the brain.
4. *Amygdala*—lays down unconscious memory (negative feelings and physical reminiscences, especially of fear events).

The amygdala often concerns us because it is the seat of the traumatic feedback loops that create posttraumatic stress disorder. But that is another story.

The religious feelings stirred by the temporal-limbic system may be akin to mystic experiences. Jeffrey L. Saver and John Rabin (1997) describe religious phenomena in this way:

> What is peculiarly distinctive to religious experience would appear, on first inspection, to reside not in the domains of affect, language, or cognition, but in perception. It is the direct sensory awareness of God or the divine that is a quintessential mark of specifically religious experience. (p. 499)

These ictal (sudden attack) events often arise unexpectedly. They are riveting and intrude on the ordinary flow of consciousness. The person experiencing such an event may simply come to a stop in whatever he or she is doing, immersed in the internal visions.

Ictal spiritual events may be accompanied by pre- or post-auras of varying emotions such as dread, joy, or awe. It is possible that the specific content of these visions may be influenced by the beliefs and reality paradigm held by the person who is experiencing an NDE.

Stephen Salloway, Paul Malloy, and Jeffrey Cummings (1997) closely link lesions in the temporal-limbic circuit to such spiritual experiences. They and other physicians (such as Saver and Rabin) identify accompanying states such as depersonalization, derealization, and dreamy states.

Depersonalization is a loss of the sense of one's own being. This state can also be recognized in mystic events where the person who is experiencing an NDE feels himself or herself become a part of all creation. He or she no longer feels that he or she is a separate person.

Derealization involves alterations in sensing one's external environment. Derealization may involve seeing a larger reality than the usual spatial (place) environment. Or it may involve seeing everything and everywhere as one (cosmic consciousness). Depersonalization and derealization are frequently encountered by very experienced, deep-level meditators. These states—and the research into them—will be discussed later in this chapter.

Yet other states await us in temporal-limbic involvement. *Dreamy states* refer to alterations of various sorts in one's state of consciousness such as may occur during a vision. Indeed, many religions seek such stages of trance. Voodoo and many ethnic religions encourage such visionary states during their rituals. Indeed, the rituals are employed to bring on the visionary states. We could trace such dreamy trance states right back to the Greek oracles at Delphi and other sites where the oracles experienced these trance states by inhaling hallucinogenic drugs.

Indeed, today's use of hallucinogenic drugs is not limited to a few oracles. Often the users of such drugs strive to produce what we might call pseudo-spiritual occasions. The point is that some states of ecstasy are seen as ultimate spiritual states.

Testing for temporal lobe ictal events reveals local changes in electrical activity at the same time that the ictal event occurs. This is not always easy to measure unless the person has frequent events. Testing can be done (1) where stimuli that initiate an event are known and can be applied in a test situation; (2) by temporarily withdrawing medications that depress ictal events; (3) in an NDE that occurs when the patient is wired to telemetry; or (4) by measurement in which a person is put under continuous EEG monitoring for several days. For some persons in whom ictal events can't be predicted, EEG measurement may be difficult to time.

Although the experience of temporal lobe visions may be seen as spiritual, the neurologist may prefer to label them as temporal lobe epilepsy.

NEAR-DEATH EXPERIENCES

The NDE is a major spiritual event after a clinical death; that is, the cessation of commonly recognized signs of life. The NDE has nothing to do with the character, hopes, or intentions of the person experiencing it. He or she may be a schoolchild or a corporate executive. He or she may be 94 or 2 years old; he or she can be afraid of his or her shadow or a bully. The NDE is typically a peak life event and potentially a life-altering one, and in almost all cases, is perceived as a spiritual event.

Medical practitioners who once ignored this phenomenon have now begun to accept and study it. The issue for many is not whether the NDE happens but what it signifies. Physicians sometimes argue that the NDE results strictly from physiological events and is unrelated to any reality beyond the body. People experiencing NDEs on the other hand, tend to feel that the experience opened their vision to a greater and deeper view of existence. A third alternative is that the experience *both* has a physiological basis and opens vision to a greater reality.

Unlike most other spiritual encounters, many NDEs take place on a medical turf, so it is not surprising that this form of spirituality is one of the most investigated. One of the early investigators, Melvin Morse (with Paul Perry, 1990) was particularly believable because his studies involved very young children who theoretically reflect less cultural bias.

Morse identified a physiological center that initiates the NDE; it rests in the Sylvian fissure of the right temporal lobe just above the ear. He reports that a group of neurologists in Chile confirmed this location. We can still wonder whether Morse and others are correct in saying right temporal lobe, or whether this might be reversed (shifted to the left temporal lobe) in a right-brain-dominant (left-handed) person.

The NDE is the most common spiritual encounter in today's world. Indeed, more than 14 million people in the United States resuscitated after being pronounced dead have brought back similar recountings, bringing this particular spiritual experience into the world of science. The accounts of so many clinically dead, resuscitated persons eventually just couldn't be ignored, even by a medical establishment that wanted nothing to do with a phenomenon that couldn't be put *under the microscope.*

Raymond Moody (1975, 1977, and 1988) was one of the first investigators to do substantial research into the NDE, conducting extensive interviews of large numbers of people with NDEs, establishing a database, and producing a comprehensive description of the NDE. Many other researchers delved into the near-death waters, for example, P. M. H. Atwater (1994) and more books by Melvin Morse with Paul Perry (1992, 1993, 2000). With modern medical resuscitation techniques, these investigators found no lack of study subjects.

ELLIS ISLAND AND THE GOOD TRIP

Researchers virtually agree on the characteristics of the NDE. The phenomenon seems to open similar doors for most people who are experiencing NDEs, although there are two types of NDEs: the good and the bad encounter. The good experiences share many characteristics, and the bad experiences have common features as well. Ironically, the good encounter gives many people experiencing NDEs a new or renewed faith in spiritual virtues, whereas the bad experience may be equally spiritual in that it gives persons undergoing it, a sense of where they may be headed. This is not to say that the many tales of descending into hell are necessarily factual; it's quite possible that the hells visited by people experiencing an NDE are of their own psychological making.

The person experiencing a good NDE may go through any number of the following aspects, but seldom all: (1) an inability to be seen or heard by the living; (2) feeling peace and painlessness; (3) having an out-of-body experience; (4) undergoing the tunnel experience—floating upward toward others, often deceased relatives and friends; (5) seeing people of light; (6) undergoing a life review; (7) rising rapidly into the heavens; (8) feeling a reluctance to return to earth; and (9) having a different sense of time and space.

Sometimes it is the atmosphere, instead of individuals, that is filled with the bright light. Indeed, people report themselves being drawn toward the bright light. The quality of the light, wherever it appears, is such that it should be too bright to be viewed, yet it can be seen without visual distress. Many returners are challenged with a *mission* to be completed during the rest of their lives.

The place most often visited during the NDE is a pleasing garden or park, a place where the vegetation is more luxurious than that on Earth, possibly psychedelic, but not especially alien. This is the *Ellis Island* of the near-death experience. Most, but not all, people experiencing an NDE go to this Ellis Island, usually populated with deceased relatives and friends. Many people experiencing NDEs have a sense that they are blocked from going too far into the perceived after-life location, as if there were a barrier which, once crossed, precludes a return to life. They either feel this or are told this by some authority on the other side.

Whom they see and the nature of the environment may be adapted to the cultural and religious beliefs of the person experiencing it. The figure of light is a good example, being seen as Jesus or another religious figure by some and as a loving nonpersonified force by others. It appears that the NDE has a universal form, but that people place different interpretations on it. Another common site is a crystal city, usually seen in the distance rather than entered. The descriptions vary somewhat; sometimes it is golden rather than crystal. In all cases, it seems to be glorious and to defy the appearance of an earthly city.

Some people with NDEs claim to return with new gifts (sometimes seen as burdens), typically psychic or energic in character. Morse (with Paul Perry, 2000) studied paranormal acquisitions of NDE returners who were identified as having been normal before their NDEs, noting that they acquired abilities such as healing cancers, seeing apparitions, developing telepathy, clairvoyance, or precognition. Some returners, Morse claimed, remain in contact with a guardian angel met during the NDE. He found paranormal abilities in one-fourth of the population in one of his NDE studies.

For example, Dannion Brinkley (with Paul Perry, 1994) says that, after an NDE, he knew what people were about to say. Additionally, he would see portions of the lives of people he was with—as if they were movies. Brinkley exhibited numerous extrasensory perceptions, but such an extensive acquisition of psychic abilities claimed by one person after an NDE is rare.

Energic changes often give these people difficulty being around machines. For example, many of them can't keep watches on their bodies running correctly. There seems to be some magnetic change in the body. This aspect of the NDE is just beginning to be researched.

The ability to channel healing energy through the hands is another example of a possible energy change. Often the emergence of such phenomena serves only to further confuse a person who has yet to integrate an NDE into his life.

Although many people are very happy to appreciate the spiritual in ordinary, day-to-day life, this linkage of the spiritual with the paranormal is an interesting one. We will find the same linkage appearing later when we look at effects of meditation.

Melvin Morse (with Paul Perry, 1992) proposes that the cause of paranormal changes in people with NDEs is a change in their electromagnetic field and electrochemical makeup. The notion that the NDE changes the electromagnetic field of a person experiencing it is not completely satisfactory as an explanatory theory because it doesn't explain *why* the electromagnetic field changes.

People with NDEs, cognizant of others' opinions, may limit what they report. Years ago, a patient who had an NDE was likely to keep it to himself so that people wouldn't think he were crazy. That still happens today with patients who have never heard of NDEs. When patients know about the phenomenon, they are likely to be more open. Unlike the predeath vision that often is reported while it is happening, the NDE is more likely to be reported later, when the patient has regained his faculties and has had more time to digest the experience.

It's now considered good medicine to let the patient know that such visions are common and that he or she is not alone. As health professionals, many of us find that, if you ask, they tell. If you don't ask, they don't tell. The trick is to ask in a way that lets the patient be free to talk about what happened, if anything, without programming him for an expected response.

After an NDE, most people return with a very positive attitude toward life. They tend to value life more than previously, they are more caring toward others, and they have no fear of death. One might say they acquire more spiritual values. This includes a major attitude change in people who were pronounced dead after a suicide attempt.

THE BAD TRIP

A small number of persons don't find themselves on Ellis Island, but in a place that is horrible. Negative NDEs don't get much press, but they do happen. Bad NDEs occur in two ways. First, some people literally feel that they descended into hell. They describe nightmarish scenes and gruesome tortures. Phillip Berman (1996) recounts a tale told to him by one interviewee who encountered a special kind of demon folk:

> They weren't trying to kill me, they were simply trying to make me hurt more. Then they began clawing at me and biting at me. And just as I'd get one off, it seemed as though five more would be back on me, clawing and pushing. (p. 88)

The theme of constant torment is common in bad trips. P. M. H. Atwater (1994) describes various hellish domains and denizens, either threatening, lifeless, or violent. Subsequently, people experiencing these negative NDEs tend to firmly believe in the existence of hell, and, not surprisingly, many change their behaviors because they don't ever want to return there.

The second type of negative NDE is not a trip to hell but a life review undergone by someone who has chronically abused others during his lifetime. In the life review, a person becomes the recipient of all the feelings of pain or pleasure that he or she has given to others. Hence, if one spent much of a lifetime inflicting physical and emotional pain on others, he or she will experience all these feelings as if they were his or her own. Dannion Brinkley (with Paul Perry, 1994), who had an NDE, says concerning his life review:

> Now, as I reviewed my life in the bosom of the Being, I relived each one of those altercations, but with one major difference: I was the receiver . . . I felt the anguish and the humiliation my opponent felt. (pp. 12–13)

Similar to those who experienced versions of hell, those undergoing a negative life review, also are motivated to change in positive ways. One can understand that the person with an NDE who led a troubled life before the experience often has the most adjustment problems. First, their selection for the experience was based solely on the fact that they died (or had a cessation of vital signs of life), with no guarantee of emotional/spiritual maturity or readiness. Indeed, an interest in spiritual matters doesn't seem to enter the equation. Hence, the person experiencing an NDE may undergo phenomena that are entirely contradictory to his or her prior belief structure. The person experiencing an NDE may be faced with the double burden of finding meaning in the NDE while simultaneously coping with an illness/injury that may have left residual bodily damage requiring physical and/or psychological rehabilitation.

Occasionally, persons not undergoing an NDE report seeing the same quality of bright light and having some portion of the NDEs. Often these are people on the brink of death, who do not actually die. Carl Jung, the psychiatrist who was once Freud's expected successor, was one of these. And the ultimate differences between his psychotherapy paradigm and Freud's are amazing. Jung gave up Freud's notion of psychosexual stages as the exclusive motivator of behavior, opting instead for a libido that could be attached to many other things, spiritual values among them.

PERSONS NOT UNDERGOING A NEAR-DEATH EXPERIENCE

Not every resuscitated, clinically dead person recounts an NDE. Many say they have no memory at all for the time during which they were clinically deceased. One could propose many different explanations for why some resuscitated, clinically deceased persons do not have an NDE. The most obvious explanation is that they simply had no such experience.

This raises the question of *degrees of death*. Even in a normal clinical death, it is difficult for medicine to set exact parameters between the living and the dead short of bodily decay. It is possible that people judged to be clinically dead have been judged on different criteria. Strange as it sounds, are some people *less dead* than others? Not every death is judged by cessation of brain function. Often, cessation of heart beat and status of the pupils are used to judge death. Given these shades of death, it would be interesting if medical parameters could be compared between people experiencing an NDE and those who don't.

REGRESSION HYPNOSIS

Alternately, it may be that clinically deceased persons who can't recount an NDE simply don't bring their experiences back with them, that they have forgotten their NDEs. Regressing the person to the death experience with hypnosis might be a useful tool in seeing if blocked memories exist for this group.

Interestingly, regression hypnosis has been used by one physician, Shakuntala Modi (2000), to regress clients back to their origins. This surprised many of her clients who found themselves, "regressed back to the time when they were one with God and there was nothing else, only God" (p. 1). As Modi states after regressing many patients and nonpatients as well:

> Consistently, my hypnotized patients claim that God does exist. They report that He always was and is, and that the universe started with God. He is the creator of everything and everybody in the universe. (p. 21)

For the reader interested in a view of creation and God through the eyes of hypnotized persons, this book is an interesting source.

MEDITATION

Meditation is another method of attempting to use the brain to reach spiritual objectives. Sanders Laurie and Melvin Tucker (1993) describe meditation as emptying of oneself:

> One closes the eyes, goes down to alpha level, and seeks the silence rather than something within or outside the self—in short, exhausting the mind as thoroughly as possible so that ideas, sounds, and sights are eliminated . . . The stilling of the mind is the goal. (p. 86)

Meditation can be further described according to the method used to reach such emptying of the self. V. Walter Odajnyk (1993) differentiates two basic methods of meditation—fixed and discursive:

> Fixed meditation aims at focusing the attention on a specific object, either internal or external . . . Discursive meditation focuses the attention on a sequence of events: for example, one of the most common religious tactics is reliving in one's imagination or through pictures the Passion of Christ; practicing some form of guided fantasy or Jung's technique of active imagination. (p. 48)

CONTEMPLATIVE ACTS

Meditation has been used as a tool in religious contemplation for centuries. Discursive meditation on Christ's *Stations of the Cross* is a common Roman Catholic example. Today, one also finds meditation used by people simply seeking more spiritual experiences. Meditation shifts one into a passive mode, cutting off the normal track of thoughts and actions. Attention is focused on the meditation object, whether it is fixed or discursive. Medically, the attempt is to circumvent left-brain control, shifting the mind away from normal everyday thought processes, away from a focus on the self. The shift is toward right-brain control, and we know that the right brain is focused on holistic thought, emotions, feelings, and even religious appreciations.

In any thought process, there is a connection between right and left sides of the brain that serves to modify thoughts (through the connecting band of fibers, the corpus callosum), so the divide between the two halves of the brain is not complete, but we are talking about dominance here. We also know that in some people the functions of the right and left sides of the brain are reversed (evidenced by the persons being left-handed).

As used here, contemplation refers to the extensive use of time in envisioning phenomena beyond one's personal life concerns. Although contemplation may take different subject matters, religious contemplation still tops the list. Alternately, a prolonged philosophic search for the meaning of life and reality might comprise a sort of contemplation, using the same right-brain-imaginative faculties. Searching for ultimate meaning, of course, might escape the specific religious label, but it still is a spiritual activity as we have defined spirituality in this book.

Whether shamanic practices are interpreted as religious or spiritual, we once again find a purposeful use of meditative states. Contemplation is used in shamanic vision quests where one seeks a vision alone in nature, concentrating on the intention of having a spiritual encounter. Sometimes decreased nourishment assists in creating such an altered state of consciousness. Shamanism also reaches this state of contemplation by a tactic that is medically called *auditory driving*. The simplest way to reach this altered state involves the rhythmic use of a drumbeat—a practice that entrains the brain waves.

Essentially, contemplation should be nonanalytic, an emptying of the mind of everything outside of the object of contemplation. Focus is placed exclusively on the subject matter of the quest.

The term, contemplation, is sometimes taken as synonymous with meditation. More often, it is seen as a special type of discursive meditation that focuses on guided visualization. Edward Maupin (1972) notes the effective use of meditation/contemplation by the Roman Catholic church, which encourages the meditator to imagine or envision what Christ, Mary, or a selected saint has experienced at a given time, during a particular event. He notes that this church has:

> . . . articulated a psychology, or map, of what happens with meditation. The conscious exercise of attention leads to a spontaneous flow of experience to which the person becomes a receptive onlooker. At its extreme, the feeling of a separate self is lost and union with the object of meditation is felt. (p. 217)

Maupin's type of contemplation is not exclusive to Roman Catholicism or Christianity, for that matter. It is used by other religions as well, each guiding the contemplative as to what he or she is to imagine. Many religions are bifurcated into two paths: (1) a primarily left-brain experience for most members and (2) a contemplative tradition practiced by a small portion of members and clergy. The first type, although primarily left-brained, can be accompanied by positive emotions, including awe and appreciation, but the thoughts and feelings arise out of what is learned and understood. The accompanying feelings are so-called normal emotions. The second path involves direct, personal experience of an envisioned sort.

Buddhism is an example of a religious or philosophic practice in which this experiential path is encouraged for all members, with meditation as its primary tool. In some religions where contemplation was primarily used by clergy in the past, the practice now is becoming popular for lay members as well.

Contemplation need not be associated with religious goals, but it usually is. For many generations, free time for contemplation was found primarily in a religious life. Even the term "contemplative" usually refers to a sequestered religious devotee. Furthermore, a religious life encourages contemplation directed beyond one's personal concerns.

For centuries, spare time was in scarce supply for the ordinary man, whereas the religious life structured time for contemplation. That is changing in much of today's Western World, where clergy find themselves responding to the increasing pressures of life like the rest of us. Alternately, today more of the laity have enough affluence to shield themselves from the daily pressures that once precluded time for contemplation. We also see an increased interest in shamanic practices as these traditions once again gain popularity. Shamanism has always involved altered states of consciousness in which the shaman is the expert. Meditation is a learned skill, and the degree to which it alters one's state of consciousness varies with the skill of the practitioner.

OTHER USES FOR MEDITATION

Medically, meditation also may be prescribed for stress reduction, lowering of blood pressure, or creating a general sense of well-being. Indeed, in modern health care institutions one often sees regular time periods set aside for patients and staff to join in meditative practices. The linkage, whether religious or health oriented, most likely is due to changes produced by meditation in brain wave frequencies. Different frequencies of brain waves are clearly associated with different levels of consciousness. Frequency ranges are separated into delta (1.5–3.5 Hz), theta (3.5–7.5 Hz), alpha (7.5–12.5 Hz), beta (12.5–20 Hz), and gamma (26–70 Hz) bands.

Study of what happens in each band is still to be refined. It is likely that some bands may be more closely connected with spiritual thoughts and feelings than others. The beta band is the most active band involved in solving problems, dealing with ordinary reality. Most people are in the beta band when awake, alert, and thinking. So this band probably has very little to do with spiritual states.

The alpha rhythm dominates in a healthy person at rest. Alpha states can include light trances. This probably is what happens when people daydream or when athletes and others get "in the flow" of an activity, where the action takes on a life and rhythm of its own, apart from the thinking direction of the brain. It seems logical that we might find spiritual feelings arising in alpha. Indeed, this is probably the level at which the beginning meditator finds himself. Alpha states may also account for why churches make such use of ritual and music or even affecting the senses by use of incense.

The theta band reflects even more diminished sensory throughput to the cerebral cortex and manifests in drowsiness or deeper trance states. Most trance states achieved by shamans, for example, are believed to be in this belt. Again, this would tie spirituality to an altered state of consciousness, certainly in shamanism, possibly in many spiritual states.

The lower delta band is often present in sleep, and we don't know a lot about it yet. It's possible that future research may show a relationship between delta bands and the mystic encounters often associated with spirituality.

Gamma waves are particularly interesting because they often occur during meditation. They are frequently called fast beta because they range from 26 to 70 Hz. They are known to result in bursts of precognition or high-level information. Here again we see the joining of high-level spiritual states and paranormal abilities.

Brain waves can now be measured by quantitative electroencephalography (QEEG), a technique that measures many more areas of brain electrical activity than traditional EEG. The QEEG and other advanced methods of studying brain activity are presently devoted to the study of persons with severe medical incapacities. Yet these techniques now exist and could be used to study spiritual states. This is not to say that all spirituality involves altered states. Yet, when most people report special spiritual moments, they tend to include a special state of mind in the recollection—and this may mean that feelings associated with spirituality employ a different brain wave state.

Radiologic studies by Andrew Newberg and Eugene D'Aquili (2001) recorded changes in brain function in meditators (Buddhist monks and Franciscan nuns) experiencing various phenomena associated with deep meditative states. Unlike Morse's studies which looked primarily at firings in the temporal lobe, Newberg and D'Aquili focused on what parts of the brain must be tuned up or tuned down to allow the mystic experience to emerge.

The centers that they identify as critical are diverse, namely, four association areas of the brain: the orientation association area, the attention association area, the verbal conceptual association area, and the visual association area. Although the brain interactions are complex, subjects who were purposefully meditating began with activation of the attention area (the frontal cortex and thalamus of the limbic system). The attention area *tuned up* as the subjects altered their usual thought patterns, attempting to eliminate all thoughts, sensations, and feelings from their minds.

This activity was followed by a tamping down of right- and left-brain orientation areas. Together, these orientation areas normally enable a person to differentiate himself from nonself and to locate himself in space. When the neural firings in these orientation areas were blunted, the meditators in this study entered various mystic states, the greatest being a total melding with reality and loss of self, that is, cosmic consciousness (Absolute Unitary Being in these authors' terms).

Altered functions in the various association areas were recorded in meditators by using single photon emission computed tomography (SPECT), a technique that reveals increased or decreased blood flow, indicative of increased or decreased activity in a given brain area. For example, SPECT consistently showed decreased activity in the meditators' orientation areas in the posterior parietal lobes.

Daniel Goleman (in dialogue with the Dalai Lama, 2004) also presents some monitoring results on a particularly advanced meditating Tibetan monk. This study used functional magnetic resonance imaging.

THE GOD GENE

Dean Hamer (2004) adds another dimension to the linkage between spirituality and physiology. He identified a specific gene, VMAT2, that enters into the complex pattern determining one's degree of spirituality. He does not claim that this is the only gene influencing one's spirituality, but it is apparently the first gene to be mapped.

As further studies amass, we may find out more about why some people are more inherently *spiritual* than others. What part does genetics play in our spirituality? Does the structure of our brain make a difference? So many questions throw us back on the old *nature or nurture* question.

SUBSTANCE ABUSE

Next we'll look at substances that are taken to stimulate (or simulate) spiritual experiences by altering brain states. Throughout time, mind-altering substances have been used by people as vehicles to reach religious or spiritual experiences. *The Diagnostic and Statistical Manual of Mental Disorders*, 4th ed. (2000), of the American Psychiatric Association lists the following 11 categories of frequently abused substances:

> . . . alcohol; amphetamine or similarly acting sympathomimetics; caffeine; cannabis; cocaine, hallucinogens; inhalants; nicotine; opioids; phencyclidine (PCP) or similarly acting arylcyclohexylamines; and sedatives, hypnotics, or anxiolytics. (p. 191)

Almost all of these substances have been used in seeking spiritual highs. We'll only look at a few of them here. Perhaps the oldest of these sources is alcohol. Bauer (1982) claimed that Alcoholic Anonymous (AA) programs succeeded because they added a spiritual element to the program. He quotes Jung as saying:

> You see, "alcohol" in Latin is *spiritus,* and you use the same word for the highest religious experiences as well as for the most depraving possession. The helpful formula is *spiritus contra spiritum.* (p. 127)

The AA program and its drug-related clone programs have always grounded recovery in a relationship to a higher power, that is, a reference to a spiritual center. Each member further defines this spiritual center in the 12-step program in his own way. Indeed, given this program, one can think of alcohol in both its usage and its cure as dealing with the spiritual.

Today, our society is awash in chemical substances that are purposely used to create altered states of consciousness. Sometimes this use is associated with a search for the spiritual; sometimes altered states are simply sought for their own sake. Vision-producing drugs can open gates on psychic and possibly mystic encounters. Hallucinogens (psychoactive drugs) are probably the most frequently used for this purpose.

Hallucinogens are drugs that alter a person's mind and mood, inducing experiences that are quite different from ordinary consciousness. They produce changes, not only in consciousness but also in perception, thought, and emotions. Essentially, they distort the way the senses work, thereby also changing perceptions of time and space. There has always been disagreement concerning what these visions ultimately mean.

Hallucinogens are divided into three types: psychedelics, dissociatives, and deliriants. Of these three categories, psychedelics are the ones most often used in seeking religious/spiritual experiences. *Psychedelics* alter cognition and perceptions and produce trance states that keep signals from everyday stimuli from reaching the conscious mind. Psychedelics can create dreamlike visions that lead to states of spiritual exhaltation. The term, psychedelic, frequently is expanded in usage to include things such as lysergic acid diethylamide (LSD) and mescalinelike actions.

Dissociatives, for example, PCP or ketamine, cause a person to dissociate from his surroundings. You will recall that earlier in this chapter Newberg and D'Aquili described a similar state produced in meditation without drugs.

Deliriants do just what the term implies, create a state of delirium (or a fuge state). This class of hallucinogens includes drugs such as atropine. Because the effects created by this class of hallucinogen can be uncomfortable, they are seldom used in seeking spiritual experiences. Some older nurses who once worked in the labor and delivery department may remember scopolamine being used to make patients in labor less aware of the pains and traumas of labor. This usage tended to distort the later memory of labor. In some ways this use might remind us of today's rohypnol, often called the date rape drug because of its ability to create anterograde amnesia, that is, to erase later memories.

Deliriants include such items as the deadly nightshade, mandrake, and other belladonna alkaloids.

New pharmacologics reach the informal and often illegal distribution channels yearly. A few of the popular hallucinogens used in raves (all-night parties featuring music, drugs, and various psychoactive experiences) presently are MDMA (Ecstasy), 4-PMA, Nexus (Afterburner), GHB (Liquid X), Ketamine (Special K), PCP (Angel Dust), Methaqualone (Ludes), and Marijuana (Grass or Weed). Today's designer drugs are frequently updated as chemistry evolves.

Similar to the NDE, the hallucinogenic drug experience does not produce phenomena merely in those prepared to integrate such experiences into their lives. There are inevitably good and bad trips, and sometimes carryover effects after the trips as well. Still, many of today's explorers court a spiritual experience, not merely a psychedelic high. If intention matters—and it may—the motivation may influence the nature of the experience that follows use of such substances.

Jeffrey L. Saver and John Rabin (1997) discuss the classic hallucinogens, LSD, psilocybin (mushrooms), and mescaline (peyote), describing effects such as vividly colored visual illusions and hallucinations, depersonalization, autoscopy (seeing oneself), euphoria, and awareness of a larger intelligence or presence. They also note that these experiences closely parallel religious and mystical experience.

Bernard Aaronson (1997) notes that each drug has its specific spectrum of effects, in thought content, emotions, perceptions of time and space, and distortions of body image. Different hallucinogens lead to different effects, and those effects can vary from situation to situation and from person to person.

The situational aspect can be recognized if one compares the context in which hallucinogens are used. Consider the present use of ecstasy (MDMA) in *raves*—where large crowds focus on psychedelic effects, including enhanced bodily sensations, often leading to multiple sexual contacts.

In contrast, the use of peyote by Native North Americans in religious gatherings tends to result in spiritual visions. The crowns of the peyote cactus (peyote buttons) contain mescaline, a very powerful hallucinogen. The use of mescaline and other ingestants has had an age-old place in the religious rituals of many tribal societies. In these instances, the purpose and use of such drugs/herbs/biologics is limited and controlled by strong cultural traditions.

Much research has been done on shamanic hallucinogens, for example, James Fadiman (1972) compares properties of Spanish Broom (*Spartium junceum*), Scotch Broom (*Cytisus scoparius*), and Canary Island Broom (*Genista canariensis*), the latter preferred by shamans for its effectiveness.

Ayahuasca, a natural Amazonian hallucinogen, may be one present choice among many people seeking mystic encounters. John Horgan (2003) describes his responses to this hallucinogen. He is convinced the drug produces authentic mystic encounters. The problem, however, is that he apparently lacks a personal reference for comparison.

Drugs used to produce (or replicate) mystic encounters are often termed *entheogenic* (God-producing) rather than hallucinogenic to illustrate the spiritual intention. Yet there is little agreement concerning the degree to which drugs actually mimic or replicate more natural mystic encounters. Nor, for that matter, can one assert just why meditation, for example, is natural whereas ayahuasca is not. Arguments abound concerning whether hallucinogenic experiences are equivalent to other mystic and spiritual encounters.

Nor are all uses of hallucinogenics recognized as such. Sharon Packer (1998) makes an interesting case for connecting mid-17th century Jewish mystical movements with outbreaks of ergot poisoning in rye breads. Ergot, of course, is a known hallucinogen.

Although natural psychoactives are still in use, the roster of manufactured hallucinogens continues to grow. LSD was one of the earliest and most researched drugs. Stansilav Grof (1988) studied LSD extensively, specifically in relation to psychic and mystic encounters, as well as exploring its place in psychotherapy. Unlike Grof, most physicians prefer not to use drugs found to have psychedelic effects. For example, the use of ketamine as an anesthestic was virtually eliminated when patients started reporting mystic encounters while under the drug.

Arthur Hastings (1972) gives an excellent description of the ever-present marijuana, known for intensifying sensations and perceptions, often with psychoactive effects. Psychotherapists often report the demotivating effects of the weed, making psychotherapy efforts futile.

There continues to be a debate concerning whether hallucinogens can lead to the same sort of experience found in nondrug-related mystic and God-seeking encounters. The question is a difficult one to answer. Can a hallucinogenic experience lead to a direct knowing concerning reality or God? Do hallucinogens have effects identical to other excitements of the spiritual centers of the brain? The answer is unclear.

Yet those of us who have served as psychotherapists to patients who have used many of these drugs often are quite aware that we may be dealing with a permanently impaired brain.

AUDITORY DRIVING

A nondrug method that humans have used to entrain the brain for thousands of years is the use of rhythmic sounds, such as the drum beat, in ceremonies designed to elicit unusual, often spiritual, experiences. A drum beat or other repetitive sound at a specific tempo can entrain an altered state of consciousness. Medically, this use of sound is called auditory driving.

The natural electrical activity of the brain is susceptible to rhythmic auditory input, whereupon brain cells begin to fire in synchrony with the beat. The effect of this auditory stimulation on the human nervous system can be that of removing the ordinary sense of reality.

The drumbeat is the most common form of auditory driving, and its origin lies in shamanic traditions. Shamanic practices, begun in preliterate tribes, continue into today's practices. Some liturgical music, for example, Gregorian chants, may employ the same tactic of modifying brain waves. Methods used to invoke auditory driving include drumming, dancing, and rhythmic sounds.

Although the drumbeat continues to be the standard in auditory driving, we might consider Robert Monroe's (1985, 1994) hemisync methods to be the high-technology equivalent. Monroe developed patterns of hemispheric synchronism by delivering selected and varied acoustic stimuli simultaneously to right and left sides of the brain. Under this auditory stimulation, a pattern of sound resolution induces prolonged altered states of consciousness in many subjects.

Auditory driving is perhaps the simplest method of inducing an altered state of consciousness and has the advantage of not introducing foreign substances into the body. It is also rapid and works successfully on large numbers of people. Different patterns of auditory driving produce different levels and different types of encounters.

SUMMARY

There is much we don't yet know about the connections between spirituality and the brain. Yet there is enough research completed to know that there are connections. So far, the main linkages have been to brain wave frequencies and altered states of consciousness, the temporal-limbic system, and to our genes. These linkages have mostly been researched in the more extreme spiritual events (e.g., meditation/NDEs).

These pathways to spiritual states, such as auditory driving, NDEs, meditative states, and hypnotic regression (not to mention the use of mind-altering drugs), all rely on creating altered states of consciousness.

Because they are extreme states, they are easier to measure than the simpler spiritual appreciations that might be acquired through a simple walk in the woods or during a church service. It is always easier to find the extreme cases first. Additionally, these are the cases that happen to fall under a medical lens. Nor has this explored all possible body/mind responses to spirituality, a subject further discussed in Chapter 4. Whatever else may be found, it is clear that there are interesting relationships between spirituality and the brain. And there are promises of more links to come as we learn more about the brain.

This chapter also looked at some of the ways in which people attempt to stimulate spiritual experiences. Some of these states, like meditation and auditory drumming, appear to be relatively harmless. On the other hand, substance abuse may not only produce some interesting spiritual or pseudo-spiritual experiences but also poses the possibility of brain damage.

Yet to return to our original question concerning the compatibility of spirituality and the brain, we might consider two things. First, the reader is referred ahead to Chapter 5 on spirituality and research. There he or she will find Wilber's (1996) model in which correlates are explained. On his model, spirituality would fall in a totally different category of phenomena than the brain, and to judge the brain and spirituality by the same evaluation method would be a research fallacy. In our society, especially in medicine, the category into which the brain falls is often credited above all other categories for phenomena. Wilber points out the error in that simple assumption.

Second, the reader might consider the point made by Newberg and D'Aquili (2001) that the brain is our access for all information of any sort as long as we are in the body. And that to give these brain-driven conclusions priority over other realities may be unreasonable. As they say, "All knowledge, then is metaphorical: even our most basic sensory perceptions of the world around us can be thought of as an explanatory story created by the brain" (p. 171).

REFERENCES

American Psychiatric Association. (2000). *The Diagnostic and Statistical Manual of Mental Disorders (DSM-IV-TR)* (4th ed., rev.). Washington, DC: Author.

Bauer, J. (1982). *Alcoholism and women.* Toronto, Canada: Inner City Books.

Berman, P. L. (1996). *The journey home: What near-death experiences and mysticism teach us about the gift of life.* New York: Pocket Books.

Brinkley, D. (with Perry, P.). (1994). *Saved by the light.* New York: Harper Paperbacks.

Carter, R. (1998). *Mapping the mind.* Los Angeles: University of California Press.

Laurie, S. G., & Tucker, M. J. (1993). *Centering: A guide to inner growth.* Rochester, VT: Destiny Books.

Maupin, E. W. (1972). On meditation. In C. T. Tart (Ed.), *Altered states of consciousness* (3rd ed., pp. 217–240). New York: HarperSanFrancisco.

Modi, S. (2000). *Memories of God and creation: Remembering from the subconscious mind.* Charlottesville, VA: Hampton Roads.

Newberg, A., & D'Aquili, E. (with Rause, V.). (2001). *Why God won't go away.* New York: Ballantine Books.

Odajnyk, V. W. (1993). *Gathering the light.* Boston: Shambhala.

Saver, J. L., & Rabin, J. (1997, Summer). The neural substrates of religious experience. *Journal of Neuropsychiatry and Clinical Neurosciences, 9*(3), 498–510.

BIBLIOGRAPHY

Aaronson, B. S. (1972). Hypnosis, depth perception, and psychedelic experience. In C. T. Tart (Ed.), *Altered states of consciousness* (3rd ed., pp. 315–323). New York: HarperSanFrancisco.

Atwater, P. M. H. (1994). *Beyond the light: The mysteries and revelations of near-death experiences.* New York: Avon Books.

Fadiman, J. (1972). Psychedelic properties of Genista Canariensis. In C. T. Tart (Ed.), *Altered states of consciousness* (3rd ed., pp. 432–438). New York: HarperSanFrancisco.

Goleman, D. (2004). *Destructive emotions: How can we overcome them? A scientific dialogue with the Dalai Lama.* New York: Bantam Books.

Grof, D. (1988). *The adventures of self-discovery.* New York: State University of New York Press.

Hamer, D. (2004). *The God gene: How faith is hardwired into our genes.* New York: Doubleday.

Hastings, A. C. (1972). The effects of marijuana on consciousness. In C. T. Tart (Ed.), *Altered states of consciousness* (3rd ed., pp. 407–431). New York: HarperSanFrancisco.

Horgan, J. (2003). *Rational mysticism: Dispatches from the border between science and spirituality.* New York: Houghton Mifflin.

Monroe, R. A. (1985). *Far journeys.* New York: Doubleday.

Monroe, R. A. (1994). *Ultimate journey.* New York: Doubleday.

Moody, R. (with Perry, P.). (1993). *Reunions: Visionary encounters with departed loved ones*. New York: Ivy Books.

Moody, R. A. (1975). *Life after life*. New York: Bantam Books.

Moody, R. A. (1977). *Reflections on life after life*. New York: Bantam Books.

Moody, R. A. (with Perry, P.). (1988). *The light beyond*. New York: Bantam Books.

Morse, M. (with Perry, P.). (1990). *Closer to the light*. New York: Villard Books.

Morse, M. (with Perry, P.). (1992). *Transformed by the light*. New York: Ballantine Books.

Morse, M. (with Perry, P.). (1993). *Reunions: Visionary encounters with departed loved ones*. New York: Ivy Books.

Morse, M. (with Perry, P.). (2000). *Where God lives: The science of the paranormal and how our brains are linked to the universe*. New York: Cliff Street Books, Harper Collins Publishers.

Packer, S. (1998). Jewish mystical movements and the European ergot epidemics. *Israel Journal of Psychiatry, 35*(3), 227–241.

Salloway, S., Malloy, P., & Cummings, J. (1997, Summer). Introduction to the neuropsychiatry of the limbic and subcortical disorders. *Journal of Neuropsychiatry and Clinical Neurosciences, 9*(3), 313–314.

Wilber, K. (1996). *A brief history of everything*. Boston: Shambhala.

CHAPTER 4

Spirituality and Psychology: Compatible or Incompatible?

Notions of spirituality today are sometimes reduced to psychological ideas. People who advance this position analyze what the brain is doing to gratify its owner rather than giving separate credence to spiritual thoughts. In a sense, this reduction of spirituality to psychology is a form of atheism quite in keeping with the so-called scientific method. Can spirituality (and religion for that matter) simply be explained away as products of human psychology? Are they merely *feel-good* prescriptions delivered by the brain much like it delivers feel-good dopamine?

In today's education, nurses often deal with spirituality through psychological models. This is a common tactic in basic nursing education as well as in psychiatric nursing. Indeed, many people assert that spiritual and religious feelings are psychological phenomena with little connection to reality. Many would say that such spiritual appreciations come about strictly through efforts to self-soothe or self-protect. In other words, religion and spirituality may be defense mechanisms for some people.

Certainly, this perspective has been dominant in the field of psychoanalysis from its inception with Freud up to today. It has a good foothold in much of medicine. Nursing has always been a mixed bag on this issue. But this question remains: Is spirituality a masked psychological variable or does it have its own substance apart from psychology?

SPIRITUALITY AS A TREATMENT FOR ILLNESS

In health care, one of the most recent influxes of spirituality and of so-called religiosity as treatment for illness started, not in nursing, but in medicine. Herbert Benson is one of the best known physicians who advocated this route.

The problem that some see with his work and the work of those who follow his suggestions is that religion and spirituality became means to another end. This shift makes spiritual and religious efforts exist, not for their own sake, but for the sake of other goals, namely good health and recovery from illness.

Even if Benson's points are valid, one must take notice when one set of values is subordinated to another—even when both sets are positive values. Take, for example, the following illustrations of Benson and Stark (1996) philosophy:

> Faith in God, however, seems to be particularly influential in healing . . . It is part of our nature to believe in an almighty power lest our health be undermined. . . . (pp. 199–200)

> According to medical research, faith in God is good for us, and this benefit is not exclusive to one denomination or theology. You can believe in God in a quiet, introspective way, or declare your convictions out loud to the world, and still reap the physiologic rewards. (p. 299)

Much of Benson's writing takes this approach: Spirituality and religion are means to the end of good health or recovery. Of course, it may be that Benson's focus on health as the end goal may simply reflect his way of convincing physicians of the importance of spirituality or religiosity. He is probably well aware that many in his intended audience have little initial interest in spirituality. By introducing spirituality and religiosity as means, not as ends, Benson avoids the necessity of taking a stand on their reality. But more recent materials by other physicians, Larry Dossey and Depak Chopra, for example, seem more balanced.

MIND AND BRAIN AS SEPARATE

One way that some authors deal with spirituality and health is to reconceptualize reality—a tactic that Benson does not employ. This enables these authors to see spirituality and health in a different context. Physicians Dossey and Chopra both propose a universal mind, apart from the brains that access it. Dossey calls this *nonlocal mind* and describes it in relation to what he labels Era III medicine (the just-beginning era, when nonlocal mind is made part of medical practice). Nonlocal mind, Dossey (1999) believes, explains many of those things that remain inexplicable when minds are seen as individual and separate (e.g., healing prayer, paranormal abilities, and intuition). He defines the nonlocal mind in this way:

> *Nonlocal* does not mean merely "a long way off" or "a very long time" but, rather, *infinitude* in space and time. If something is nonlocal it is *unlimited*. Nonlocality, like pregnancy, is an all-or-nothing event. (p. 26)

In addition to nonlocal mind being everywhere and unlimited, Dossey claims that it is fundamental in nature that it cannot be divided into more basic components.

Chopra (2000) makes a claim similar to Dossey's. In differentiating between mind and brain, he sees brain as a bodily vehicle and mind as a greater entity that can't be located in space–time and certainly can't be located in brain tissue. The mind is a field into which one taps rather than a confined organ; mind is greater than mere biology. Chopra proposes a universal *mind field*, which one accesses. Here, Chopra describes a phenomenon (brain), not by reference to its smaller parts, but by reference to its participation in something greater (mind).

In differentiating mind and brain, Chopra's perception of mind is much like Dossey's. Chopra suggests a shared, universal mind field, a domain that individuals tap with differing degrees of ability. Chopra specifically asserts that mind equates with God. Regardless of whether one states this as a conclusion, clearly this sort of philosophy places meaning in a higher realm. As Chopra (2000) says:

> Our whole notion of reality has actually been topsy-turvy. Instead of God being a vast, imaginary projection, he turns out to be the only thing that is real, and the whole universe, despite its immensity and solidity, is a projection of God's nature. (p. 2)

For Chopra, the brain is our way of entering the mind. If *all knowing* is derived from the universal mind, that is, God, then from Chopra's perspective, some people simply tap into more of the field than others.

Conceptualizing mind in this form of dialectic is one way that spirituality is reentering the world of medical care. This is a major revision in a profession long wedded to a third-person reductionist perception of reality.

Goswami (with Reed and Goswami, 1993) express a similar idea in relation to quantum physics, proposing that a change in philosophic perspective from material realism to idealism makes sense of the quantum physics view of the world (as opposed to the older Newtonian one):

> . . . mind and matter are integrally part of one reality because ideas . . . and the consciousness of them are considered to be the basic elements of reality; matter is considered to be secondary. (p. 10)

HISTORICAL RELATIONSHIPS OF ILLNESS AND SPIRITUALITY

Many disciplines have contributed in linking illness and spirituality, often using different conceptualizations from those of Dossey and Chopra. For example, beginning with the assertions of the famous psychic and mystic Emanuel Swedenborg (George Dole, 1979, 1984), several investigators of the hallucinations of psychotic patients have identified universal patterns for the phenomena reported by patients *possessed* by demons or speaking with angels. In other words, different patients, not in contact with each other, describe these demons and/or angelic beings in remarkably similar ways.

Psychiatrist Wilson Van Dusen (1974) carried out systematic enquiries at Mendocino State Hospital, building descriptions of two worlds, those of the low spirits and those of the high ones. Similar to Swedenborg's assertions, when psychotic patients were asked to describe these worlds, they reported virtually identical phenomena, that is, identical characteristics shared among these patients' demonic and angelic beings, specifics that could not all be traced to common legends and folklore.

D. Scott Rogo (1987) reached similar findings concerning the worlds of the lower spirits. If such visions were truly isolated in the mind of each patient, such corresponding findings would be astounding. If these interpretations of shared demonic and angelic worlds have any validity, we might say that a psychosis occurs when someone inadvertently opens a door into another dimension and is unable to close it.

Notice the philosophic difference here. Where Chopra, for example, connected the medical and spiritual at a higher level (universal mind field), Van Dusen and Rogo see spiritual or religious elements (demons or angels) as infringements on the patient's psyche. Yet works of Van Dusen and Rogo point to a world that is separate from each patient's brain, a world that is shared among patients/people. In a sense, this sort of study gives backup to claims that spiritual realms have some existence outside of psychology and outside of individual brains. At least that would be one possible interpretation.

Of course, the studies of this sort are unusual in that they actually look at patients' worlds without prejudging them as invalid (merely in the mind). R. H. Prince and Margaret Reiss (1990) claim that this is an unusual response. The typical reaction of the psychiatrist, so they say, is to dismiss the patient's world as delusional, paying little attention to the content of the expressed ideas:

> In dismissing these ideas as meaningless, the psychiatrist relegates highly significant experiences of the patient to limbo . . . For the psychiatrist, the explanatory model (EM) of the patient with respect to his or her experience is completely unrealistic and even more damaging, non-negotiable. (p. 141)

Views such as those of Swedenborg, Van Dusen, Rogo, and Prince and Reiss grant that different perceived worlds deserve our attention. And these different perceived worlds, good or bad, may have spiritual/religious origins and significance.

Are spiritual domains different from psychological ones? Are they associated? Do altered states of consciousness open doors to different realities? Do multiple doors exist? Do alternate worlds coexist? For example, does the shaman's world coexist with the Ellis Island of the newly deceased as revealed in near-death experiences (NDEs), or with the world of hierarchical souls as described by Robert Monroe (1994) and by Michael Newton (1994, 2002). Monroe's group reaches this information by using hemisynch auditory manipulations to produce altered states of consciousness (different sound patterns delivered to each of the ears). Newton uses hypnotic regression of clients to life between lives.

Newton (1994) reports that souls are organized in the spirit world after death:

> . . . a soul's journey back home ends with debarkation into the space reserved for their own colony, as long as they are not a very young soul or isolated for other reasons. . . . The souls represented in these cluster groups are intimate old friends who have about the same awareness level. (p. 87)

Newton gives much more content concerning the world encountered between lives in his more recent (2004) book. Again, the information was collected by use of hypnotic regression on large numbers of clients.

Monroe, using his technique of hemisynch-induced trance for his subjects/investigators, reports finding similar afterlife groups of like-level souls. He also tells of finding groups whose members have created *heavens* that meet their religious expectations. Apparently, there is accommodation for those who die with rigidly held beliefs. Members of these groups report to Monroe's investigators that now and then a member just *disappears* never to return again. Monroe's investigators believe that this happens when a member realizes that this created heaven is illusory, and they move on to less imaginary realms.

Can these other realities offer special knowledge concerning an overarching reality supporting all these possibilities? The shaman's world, the afterlife world, and the demonic–angelic worlds represent only a few potentials.

History is replete with examples that suggest the possibility of multiple worlds. And many of these worlds have spiritual implications. Maybe today's certitude concerning the scientific worldview isn't a function of increased wisdom but is instead an increased locking of the doors between worlds. If we truly live in an era when there is a shift concerning what comprises reality, then perhaps a few of the alternate doors are being pushed ajar. Indeed, doors are an apt analogy for these portals between worlds.

Whether one believes in an afterlife or not, it is interesting that different researchers find similar realms between lives, while using different methods to arrive at these conclusions. It is also interesting that both Newton's subjects and Monroe's subjects/researchers identify reincarnation as a fact underlying this system.

THE PSYCHIATRIC NURSE AND PSYCHOTHERAPY

Nursing has an interesting history with psychotherapy. Originally, most nurses interested in psychotherapy assumed that they would work in psychiatric settings. One of the first nursing theories to surface was one for psychiatric nursing created by Hildegard Peplau (1952). Her theory was modeled on Harry Stack Sullivan's (1953) *interpersonal relationship* theory. For many years, Peplau's nursing adaptation took precedence in most nursing psychiatric programs.

In Sullivan's theory, the human becomes social at birth. He or she must be understood based on his network of interpersonal relationships; he or she is culturally imbedded. Focus is placed on the I–You interactions by which the person assumes that certain behaviors will elicit certain reactions. These so-called *parataxic integrations* can become rigid and dominate the person's thinking patterns, leading to major distortions. In Sullivan's interpersonal school of psychoanalysis, such problems in living are the focus, and the therapist interacts with the patient to make these distortions evident and then to help the patient change them.

Briefly, Peplau's interpersonal relationship theory focused on four phases in the nurse–client relationship:

1. *Orientation*—nurse and patient collaborate in a reciprocal process of analyzing the problem and getting beyond being strangers.
2. *Identification*—patient responds to the help offered either independently, interdependently, or dependently; as the interrelationship with the nurse advances, the patient gains a sense of competency.
3. *Exploitation*—patient takes advantage of all available services, essentially increasing his control of the situation through resource selection and management.
4. *Resolution*—the patient's needs have been met through the nurse–patient relationship and the links between them must be terminated successfully, freeing the patient to move on.

Today, interpersonal relationship theory (in relation to either Sullivan or Peplau) is seldom the approach of choice in psychotherapy. Other theories have assumed dominance in the field.

The roles of nurses in mental health have also changed. Many now have private psychotherapy practices rather than working with psychiatric inpatients. Indeed, development of psychiatric nurse practitioner programs occurred very early in the development of nurse practitioner roles. Because many of these programs occur at the master's level today, it is often the case that such programs select one therapeutic path rather than providing an eclectic education in psychological theories. Presently, some of those programs design a specific curriculum for nurses and others select a psychotherapeutic theory shared with other professions. Cognitive therapy (CT) (Beck, Rush, Shaw, & Emery, 1979) and cognitive behavioral therapy (CBT) (e.g., Linehan, 1993), for example, present techniques that can be nicely honed within the length of a master's program.

Many present psychological theories could be called spiritually neutral or negative. However, the National Organization of Nurse Practitioner Faculties (2002) has included the spiritual in their document, *Domains and Core Competencies of Nurse Practitioner Practice.* The spiritual competencies include (but are not limited to) assisting patients and families meet spiritual needs and assessing the influence of the patient's spirituality on health care practices.

Once again (as we found in Chapter 2 with NANDA's nursing diagnoses), we find a pattern whereby nurses are held accountable for achieving goals concerning which they have little education and probably less assessment talent than might be required.

TRADITIONAL PSYCHOTHERAPEUTIC MODELS

Many traditional psychotherapeutic models have been used in nursing education. Briefly and incompletely we might start with Sigmund Freud in the late 19th century. Freud's (e.g., 1962) basic theory elements usually are taught even in the psychiatric component of nursing bachelor's programs. The focus in this and other developmental theories is on childhood, although problems can occur anywhere along the line. The therapist helps the client recognize these old patterns and how they are carrying forward in time to cause problems in the present life.

Drive Theory

Freud's theory is a drive theory because in it, the human being is born with innate drives/instincts that bring about other significant processes. Freud's drives (urges) are the instigators of human response, and they are focused around infantile serial stages of sexuality:

1. *Oral* phase—drives are focused on the mouth and oral mucosa. Oral fixations may include addictions, eating disorders, or obesity.
2. *Anal* phase—drives are focused on the anus with the infant retaining or letting go of the products of the bowel (18 months–2 years). Anal fixations may result in excessive orderliness or obstinacy.

3. *Aphallic/genital* phase—drives have a penile focus (age 2–3). Before this time, children don't notice there's a difference between the sexes.
4. *Genital* phase—drives focus on the genitalia (3½–5 years) and genital pleasure.
5. *Oedipal* stage—drive usually relates to the desire for exclusivity with opposite-sex parent, contesting (or wishing to contest with) the same-sex parent.

Other important Freudian principles include the *Ego*, *Id*, and *Superego*. The id carries the drives/urges, whereas the superego carries the super conscience. The ego is the arbitrator of the system. But for Freud the ego was merely the rider on the back of the id. Freud needed some in-born learning and adaptation structure, but he did not give the ego the attention it received from later theorists.

Freud's goal was drive satisfaction (the pleasure principle). His theory also required negotiation with the reality principle. Because he lived in an era of much social repression, he had many references to the building of a conscience. Freud wanted the human being to be totally describable and predictable, with everything going back to drive satisfaction or frustration.

After Freud, most theories built on (or competed with) his theory, each emergent theory seeing the human being as more and more complex. Interestingly, each theory made the infant less a creature of drives and more a creature who comes into the world with *more in place*.

Freud was an atheist, and this belief permeated his theory. It also set the scene for many psychotherapists to follow. This holds even today.

Ego Theory

In *ego theory*, Anna Freud (1946), Heinz Hartmann (1958), and others claimed that the personal organization was more than the mere expression of drives (although they did not question that such drives existed). But they saw the Freudian sexual phases more like periods of critical formative events, of separation/individuation. They noted that childhood has rapid development and that regularly recurring moments of tension (like needing to move bowels, eat, learning to speak, conceptualizing *mama*, saying *no*, pulling the self up in crib, or learning to walk) lead to a personal psychology, fantasies, and sublimations.

These new abilities bring joys as they emerge. Growth and development is not just drive satisfaction in ego theory. The child experiences his own efficacy, not just at critical moments but also during recurring calm moments. The child builds a defense organization and learns adaptation and reality testing. The goal in ego theory is for the child to develop autonomy and efficacy, and this requires the confirmation of others for the development to occur.

Hence, ego theory did not challenge the elements of Freud's theory but simply added on elements of adaptation. It clearly, however, was shifting away from the previous singular importance of Freud's sexual stages of growth.

Object Relations Theory

Object relations theory claims that what matters most is the person's relationships with objects. These *objects* are often people (or parts of people—like the breast in infancy). This theory can be represented by Melanie Klein (1975) and Donald W. Winnicott (1971), who are even farther away from Freud than ego theory.

Object seeking, not pleasure/satisfaction seeking, is the goal here. It's not all intense intrusions (e.g., drives), not just satisfaction of a momentary drive. The person's life is of his own making (including his wishes, fantasies, and character development), not just what drives occur.

The person is an entity with a constitutional capacity for love and destructive impulses. He or she learns to internalize the objects—good ones and feared ones. He or she introjects objects into himself or herself, and they become part of who he or she is. His or her intimate caretakers are examples of objects usually internalized.

Winnicott extends this notion of introjection into transitional objects for the child (it's not just a teddy bear or a blanket). For example, the child can do without the mother for a while because he or she has introjected her into the safety of the blanket.

The goal in object relations is the joy (or by default, the trauma) of object-related experience.

Self Theory

Heinz Kohut developed this theory centered on the self (Kohut & Wolf, 1978), which crystallizes in interplay of inherited and environmental factors and then aims toward realizing its own program. This theory adds a native creativity—and we're now a long way from Freud.

To crystallize the self, the child needs *mirroring* (parroting back to the child his greatness—(mirrored grandiosity) and *idealizing* by others. Gradually self objects are replaced with a self (about age 2). Self constituents include:

1. A pole of basic strivings for power and success
2. A pole for basic idealized goals
3. Talents and skills activated by the tensions between the two poles

The goal of the child is a program of action determined by these three factors. The therapy under self theory is different than others in that the therapist's supportiveness takes precedence over the patient gaining insight. The person learns empathy for himself. The goal of self theory is to build and maintain self-esteem. This program adds self-driving to creativity. Notice how each new theory adds other dimensions of humanness beyond Freud's conceptualization of drives.

All of the above theories explore the past to understand the present (usually adulthood) except Kohut's self theory, where amelioration or cure of the central disturbance, not suppression or understanding of symptoms, is what counts most.

Carl Jung

Many of Freud's followers tried their wings by substituting something other than his innate drives as the engine of the system—for example, Adler's (1958) notion of power as the dominant moving force. Freud had no tolerance for those who wanted to make changes in his model. His heir apparent, Carl Jung (1963, 1971), eventually exemplified this conflict with the master.

Jung expanded Freud's notion of libido beyond just the sexual arena, conceiving of it as psychic energy attached to interests, attention, and drives (value-charged individual drives, not just Freud's sexual ones). Jung truly created a new theory. The nurse will recognize many of his basic elements:

Persona—one's public face

Anima—female soul in the male

Animus—male soul in the female

Shadow—the unconscious part of the personality with weaknesses one's self-esteem won't recognize as one's own

Synchronicity—an acausal connecting principle—meaningful coincidences

Archetype—universal and recurring images/motifs of typical human experiences emerging from the collective unconscious, possibly in dreams/visions; a transpersonal power that transcends the ego

Collective unconsciousness—the deepest unconscious layer, suprapersonal, ordinarily inaccessible

Ego—the sum of individual's experience of subjective identity

Introversion—interest and value attached to inner life

Extraversion—interest and value attached to external objects

Jung had many spiritual appreciations attached to his thoughts and his notions of reality. Indeed, it is likely he underwent a near-death encounter himself. These spiritual appreciations, of course, clashed greatly with Freud's avowed atheism and his notion of science. Indeed, Freud's atheism has had a long-lasting effect, even on psychotherapists of our time.

These are just a few examples of theories of the human being that arose after Freud. Notice that most of them use the same methodology. They reach into the past to find the patterns (and the reasons for the patterns) that explain the present difficulties. One could say that they bring right-brain problems (emotional) to the left brain and analyze them in order to overcome them.

Alternately, some later psychotherapy deals with the same emotional problems by keeping them in the right brain, but modifying them there emotionally instead of analytically. This is done when the client, for example, is asked to relive the emotion with a different imagined ending. With this tactic, one sees such things as the client invited to beat up a pillow as if it were the childhood abuser, to display the invective that could not be expressed in the original situation. See, for example, Roger Woolger's (2004) exploration of past lives.

For some patients, reliving a trauma (perhaps with a different ending) may be a useful tactic; for others it will not. Nor is it useful in all situations. For example, just reliving a trauma severe enough to engender PTSD can deepen the trauma.

In general, the psychotherapist operates with what is usually termed evenly suspended attention to the expressed thoughts of the patient. And those thoughts are usually produced through free association. When appropriate, the therapist gives a careful interpretation of what the patient is saying. This helps him give meaning to the previously veiled connections.

Cognitive Therapy and Cognitive Behavioral Therapy

Aaron Beck et al. (1979) originated a new method of psychotherapy that acts by a different mechanism. CT brings misconceptions for left-brain analysis and treatment, but it remains in the here and now, not in the past. The focus is on *present* thoughts that represent distorted conclusions that the client holds. The client is encouraged to bring these distortions to the logical analysis and testing capacities of the left brain. The system doesn't deal with when, where, or under what circumstances the distortion arose. The objective is to change the distortions in the present by directly testing their veracity in the client's present world.

In this form of therapy, the psychotherapist is much more interactive than usual. The therapist points out the presumed distortions and helps the client challenge his perceptions by designing altered behaviors for the client to test in the interval before his next appointment. The therapy is based on a contract between the therapist and client as the crux of treatment. The client is given assignments between visits to the psychotherapist, and the assignments, if followed, test the distortions, allowing the patient to discover for himself the flaws in his reasoning.

Because this approach arose in an era when behaviorism was popular, some therapists prefer CT to CBT notions to make certain their processes are differentiated from this other method. (Behaviorism stressed that the simple altering of behavior would subsequently alter the associated thought processes—with the operation of cognitive dissonance as the driving force.) Clearly, however, the altered thought patterns resulting from CT have the potential for changing behaviors as well as thoughts. But the change, unlike behaviorism, results from the new cognitive understanding.

One can see that CT and/or CBT have a certain charm for master's programs in nursing because they are highly formulated. Hence, they can be mastered in the relatively short time of a master's program. Although learning the process may be quicker for the therapist than other methods, the results also may be rather more rapid for the patient than other methods. Indeed, when Beck originated this therapeutic intervention, he was driven to find a system that showed quicker results than traditional psychotherapy.

The difference between CT/CBT and older methods, then, is one of (1) time—most of the analysis deals with present thought patterns; and (2) the degree of intervention by the therapist—greatly enhanced and contractual, using defined protocols that require patient–professional agreed-upon interventions.

One might note some of the reasons why CT/CBT has appeal today as compared to Freudian analysis. Freud's method of psychoanalysis occurred in a different era. He would see patients five to six times a week, and the time allotted for analysis was not limited by insurance standards. Today, this process would be extremely expensive, as virtually no insurance plan would pay for such intensive therapy.

Further, Freud self-selected a specific type of patient, basically wealthy neurotics who didn't have problems with a basic underlying sense of self. Freud refused, for example, to analyze schizophrenics. And he did not deal with clients who exhibited ego function defects or ego/self-deficits, let alone those with object relations failures. His practice was unique, not competitive, and he could exclude patients with these flaws. Today's psychotherapists don't have the luxury of limiting their practice to Freud's preferred patients. Indeed, the psychological problems of our era are quite different as is the patient mix of diagnoses.

SUMMARY

When we look at any of these methods of psychotherapy, they may be seen as neutral at best in regard to spirituality. Yet the tradition, beginning with Freud, is for many therapists to approach their work from a position of atheism. This is not so in all cases, however. See, for example, the work of the Association for Spirituality & Psychotherapy (a group of psychotherapists from diverse educational backgrounds). Indeed, the group members include many nurse psychotherapists.

Can spirituality, and religion for that matter, simply be explained away as products of human psychology? It is clear that many psychotherapists take this stance. But we have identified some patterns that draw upon spirituality within psychology. First we have argued from metaphysics: a dialectic movement from matter to spirit, that is, from brain to nonlocal mind. We also find movements recommending alternate states of consciousness as vehicles to reach alternate worlds, many with spiritual/religious elements.

Over history, we can see definite trends—with some modern therapy sacrificing scientific and materialistic worldviews to worldviews incorporating spiritual values. Still, we find the strong atheistic influence of Freudian analysis.

In nursing, some but not all, holistic programs incorporate spiritual elements in psychotherapy. And much of our literature assumes that nurses have responsibility for achieving spiritual goals.

Can spirituality be reduced to psychology? We find mixed answers at the moment with contradictory trends. Yet we find more and more systems of psychotherapy giving credence to spirituality as its own domain, with its own reality.

REFERENCES

Benson, H., & Stark, M. (1996). *Timeless healing: The power and biology of belief.* New York: Simon & Schuster (Fireside Book).

Chopra, D. (2000). *How to know God: The soul's journey into the mystery of mysteries.* New York: Harmony Books.

Dossey, L. (1999). *Reinventing medicine: Beyond mind-body to a new era of healing.* San Francisco: HarperSanFrancisco.

Goswami, A. (with Reed, R. E., & Goswami, M.). (1993). *The self-aware universe: How consciousness creates the material world.* New York: Jeremy P. Tarcher/Putnam.

Newton, M. (1994). *Journey of souls.* St. Paul, MN: Llewellyn Publications.

Prince, R. H., & Reiss, M. (1990). Psychiatry and the irrational: Does our scientific world view interfere with the adaptation of psychotics? *Psychiatric Journal of the University of Ottawa, 15,* 137–143.

BIBLIOGRAPHY

Adler, A. (1958). *What life should mean to you.* New York: Capricorn Books.

Beck, A. T., Rush, A. J., Shaw, B. F., & Emery, G. (1979). *Cognitive therapy of depression.* New York: Guilford Press.

Dole, G. F. (Ed. & Trans.). (1979). *Swedenborg's heaven and hell.* New York: The Swedenborg Foundation.

Dole, G. F. (Ed. & Trans.). (1984). *Emanuel Swedenborg: The universal human and soul-body interaction.* New York: Paulist Press.

Freud, A. (1946). *The ego and the mechanisms of defence* (C. Baines, Trans.). New York: International Universities Press.

Freud, S. (1962). *Three essays on the theory of sexuality* (J. Strachey, Ed. & Trans.). USA: Basic Books.

Greenberg, J., & Mitchell, S. (1983). *Object relations in psychoanalytic theory.* Cambridge, MA: Harvard University Press.

Hartmann, H. (1958). *Ego psychology and the problem of adaptation* (D. Rapaport, Trans.). New York: International Universities Press.

Jung, C. (1971). *The portable Jung.* USA: Penguin Books.

Jung, C. G. (1963). *Memories, dreams, reflection: C. J. Jung (rev. ed.).* In A. Jaffe (Ed.) and R. Winston & C. Winston (Trans.). New York: Vintage Books.

Klein, M. (1975). *Love, guilt and reparation.* New York: The Free Press.

Kohut, H., & Wolf, E. (1978). The disorders of the self and their treatment: An outline. *International Journal of Psychoanalysis, 59,* 413–425.

Linehan, M. M. (1993). *Cognitive-behavioral treatment of borderline personality disorder.* New York: Guildford Press.

Monroe, R. A. (1994). *Ultimate journey.* New York: Doubleday.

Monroe, R. A. (1985). *Far journeys.* New York: Doubleday.

National Organization of Nurse Practitioner Faculties. (2002). *Domains and core competencies of nurse practitioner practice.* Washington, DC: Author.

Newton, M. (2002). *Destiny of souls: New case studies of life between lives.* St. Paul, MN: Llewellyn Publications.

Newton, M. (2004). *Life between lives: Hypnotherapy for spiritual regression.* St. Paul, MN: Llewellyn Publications.

Peplau, H. E. (1952). *Interpersonal relations in nursing.* New York: G. P Putnam's Sons.

Rogo, D. S. (1987). *The infinite boundary: A psychic look at spirit possession, madness and multiple personality.* New York: Dodd, Mead & Company.

Sullivan, H. S. (1940). *Conceptions of modern psychiatry.* New York: W. W. Norton & Co.

Sullivan, H. S. (1953). *The interpersonal theory of psychiatry.* New York: W. W. Norton & Co.

Van Dusen, W. (1974). *The presence of other worlds.* New York: Harper & Row.

Winnicott, D. W. (1971). *Playing and reality.* New York: Basic Books.

Woolger, R. (2004). *Healing your past lives: Exploring the many lives of the soul.* Boulder, CO: Sounds True.

CHAPTER 5

Spirituality and Research: What Research Makes Sense? What Doesn't?

This chapter challenges much of the present research that claims to investigate spirituality. The challenge deals with the nature of the research applied to the subject matter of spirituality. This chapter, then, serves as a caution against the most common error in research into spirituality: a mismatch of subject matter and method of research.

Most contemporary studies of spirituality and/or religion use research tools with quantitative measurements. It's true we can count how many people attend church and how many people claim to have fewer symptoms in groups matched on religion/no religion categories. Of course, it's a lot easier to list people by religion than to try to separate them on spirituality. (See Chapter 1 if you need to be reminded about this complexity.)

Yes, there are a lot of things we can count and lots of demographic and census data we can collect. But do these collections really deal with spirituality itself? I'm suggesting that spirituality itself can't be captured with this sort of certainty. Spirituality is complex and different for every person. Spirituality deals with what has ultimate meaning for an individual, and we're all different. The following material explains this common mismatch between subject matter and research.

Before we do research on *any* topic, we'd do well to look at its nature. What kind of concepts or constructs comprise it? What are we hoping to investigate? Our phenomenon is *spirituality:* a very complex notion.

Spirituality relates to one's conception of the whole world and all of existence. Our sense of the spiritual tells us what we conceive to be the underlying nature of reality, how things are in the universe. It tells us how we are in the world and what moves us to care about the universe and the people and the things in it. Spirituality deals with those values we hold most dear.

Spirituality involves the mysteries and subtleties of life. These questions don't lend themselves so easily to operational terms and head counts. Indeed, the very nature of spirituality clashes with our present desire for certainty. This is especially true during nursing's present focus on quantitative research.

When we really want to research spirituality, we need to ask two essential questions. First, the ontological one: In what kind of world does this research make sense? What view of the world makes the research question logical? In what kind of reality will the research question tell us something about our subject matter? And next, we need to ask the epistemological question: How do we know that what we know is valid?

Suppose we do a survey which tells us that churchgoers get fewer postoperative symptoms than nonchurchgoers after a given surgical procedure. That tells us something about healing, but it doesn't tell us anything directly about spirituality itself.

The problem is a mismatch between the research method and the subject matter. Whether we like it or not, spirituality is a phenomenon that lends itself most readily to qualitative research, not quantitative.

Ken Wilber (1996) notes that we can examine any phenomenon from four different positions. He calls these the *Four Quadrants of the Kosmos*. They are essentially four different lenses through which we can view any subject matter. He describes these positions in the following manner.

INTERIOR	EXTERIOR
UPPER LEFT	UPPER RIGHT
"I"	"IT"
INTENTIONAL	*BEHAVIORAL*
SINGULAR	*SINGULAR*
(Subjective-intentional)	(Objective-behavioral)
INTERIOR	EXTERIOR
LOWER LEFT	LOWER RIGHT
"WE"	"ITS"
CULTURAL	*SOCIAL*
PLURAL	*PLURAL*
(Cultural-intersubjective)	(Interobjective-social)

FIGURE 5.1   Wilber's Four Quadrants of the Kosmos

The left-hand side of his quadrant contains two sections, both taking an interior viewpoint (seen from inside the viewer or researcher). He abbreviates the upper left quadrant as the *I* (singular) focus, while the lower left-hand side is the *we* (plural) position. Both the singular and plural quadrants report how the phenomenon is experienced.

The right-hand side of his four quadrants takes an exterior viewpoint (the phenomenon is separate from the viewer or researcher). He labels the top quadrant the *it* (singular) box while the lower becomes the *its* (plural) location. Here again, the singular and the plural are differentiated. Hence the four quadrants give all the options of combining the singular and the plural with positions interior and exterior to the researcher. Wilber's quadrants form a map in which to locate any phenomenon.

Yet an interesting thing happens when a phenomenon is distributed among any of these positions: the phenomenon changes radically in each quadrant. As illustration, *mind* might be a phenomenon in the upper left-hand corner (interior, singular). I perceive my *mind*; I know what I'm thinking. But if I skip over to the right-hand quadrant, I no longer find mind; instead I find *brain*. Mind is felt internally, brain is seen from the outside.

The quadrant addressing the mind involves intention, whereas the quadrant witnessing brain is behavioral. I see the behavior of the subject's brain but I don't perceive it directly. Or we could go further and recognize *self* and *consciousness* on the left side while *neocortex* might form the

UPPER LEFT	UPPER RIGHT
Mind	Brain
Self and consciousness	Neocortex
Perceptual states	Limbic system
Intentions	Molecules, atoms
Freud, Carl Jung, Buddha	B. F. Skinner, John Locke
Phenomenology	Empiricism
LOWER LEFT	LOWER RIGHT
Culture	Social systems
Magic, myth	Ethnic tribes, feudal empires
Hermeneutics	Systems theory

FIGURE 5.2   Wilber's Four Quadrants of the Kosmos—Some Examples

right-side equivalent. Again, notice that the phenomenon has radically changed.

In the lower plural quadrants, we might compare viewpoints of a culture on the left-hand side—how it feels to be a member of a given group, while the right-hand side (the external plural) could be labeled social—what I see when I observe a group, perhaps as an anthropologist.

Notice that none of Wilber's four lenses can be reduced to one of the others. Later Wilber (2007) realized that from a research perspective, these viewpoints could be further divided into eight different orientations, but we don't have to go that far to make the point that phenomena correspond but change depending on the quadrant from which they are viewed. And when we look at a phenomenon, we had best recognize the quadrant in which it fits, because the nature of the quadrant will suggest legitimate methods of research for that location.

Wilber's differentiations would suggest that, where people try to reduce aspects of mind—let's say a thought—to brain, perhaps the parts of the brain activated on functional magnetic resonance imaging (fMRI), they are simply wrong. A thought: *I'm going to kill my spouse*—cannot be reduced to a spot (or spots) on the brain that light up in an fMRI. That's something different. To try to reduce any of the four corners to one of the other is a false reductionism. They correspond, Wilber says, but they are not identical.

When we look at spirituality, it is clear that it is much more like mind than like brain. It is an inferred perception, a concept that would belong in Wilber's upper left quadrant (when speaking as an individual or lower left quadrant if one were asserting a shared spirituality within a group).

NURSING AND LOGICAL POSITIVISM

Wilber's schema makes us think back about nursing's long and misplaced love affair with Logical Positivism. When major nursing groups decided that nursing should make moves to become a profession and an academic field (beginning in the early 50s), the world was in the grasp of a research philosophy called Logical Positivism. This system was essentially discredited in its own field of philosophy by 1969. Yet it lingered in nursing for many years thereafter. Of course, it is not unusual when disciplines that borrow ideas from other fields keep the borrowed ideas longer than the initiating field.

Logical Positivism espoused that there was only one way of doing research that was valid: classical empirical research (quantitative method with hypothesis testing, control groups—the usual testing methods applied today in empirical research). At its inception, Logical Positivism was seen as the *only* acceptable route to knowledge. It was touted as the only answer to the epistemological question for *any* subject matter.

There are, of course, circumstances where this model works very well, for example, researching a disease caused by an organism that attacks the cells. Indeed, many research questions that have uniform answers for all comers operate in this fashion. In other words, this research method is perfectly compatible with Wilber's upper right-hand quadrant.

The problem was that the advocates of Logical Positivism thought that *all* scientific disciplines could be researched by the same method. Let me give you a negative example of what happened: Sigmund Freud, who began his work when Logical Positivism was in bloom, wanted to be the consummate scientist when formulating his theories, identifying, for example, elements that today we call ego, id, and superego. And he attempted to *prove* the existence of these components by the rules of Logical Positivism.

The easiest way to see his error is to say that no one ever saw an id, ego, or superego on autopsy. Freud failed to recognize the difference between *empirical, material* components and *conceptual* components. One can't say an ego or an id is either *real* or *unreal*. Freud's terms are ways of seeing and interpreting actions and reported feelings. Today, we would say these are qualitative elements (Wilber's upper left quadrant).

The limitation (or the beauty, if you prefer) of qualitative terms is that someone else can come along and explain the same phenomenon with a different set of concepts having different labels. In qualitative research, a conceptual framework lasts as long as it is the most coherent and useful explanation of a phenomenon. In the case of Freud's system, for example, it has been replaced (by some) with systems such as Jung's theory, object relations, or self-psychology, among many other explanatory construct schemas. And there is not one-to-one matching of such competing systems. Jung's *shadow,* for example, is not identical to Freud's id.

MANAGING DIFFERENT SORTS OF PHENOMENA

The flaw in a unitary notion of research is that one method (such as Logical Positivism) simply won't fit all subject matters. The research method, if it is to be valid, must be in synchrony with the nature of its subject. The first step in looking at the fit between the research method and its target is to know the subject matter (phenomenon) intimately. In our case, we want to research spirituality itself, not its correlates in the other quadrants.

Hence, we have to know the nature of that subject matter before we can figure out what research methods are compatible. There are several steps we can take in order to do that.

First, we can look at a phenomenon from its four chief elements:

1. *Content*: the meat of the matter, the most important concepts.
2. *Process*: what makes the system move, the action principle; the method of thinking or acting.
3. *Context*: the nature of the world being considered; the background of the phenomenon (like water would be the context for the fish).
4. *Goal*: the end point, the aim of the system; the objectives, whether they have been identified in advance or not).

On these dimensions we might say about spirituality that:

1. It deals with ultimate perceived values (content).
2. Felt emotions, motivated by thoughts about what is meaningful, derive the values (process).
3. Spirituality occurs in a world where meaning can be ascribed, and some elements have more significance than others (context).
4. One recognizes which values are more important in one's life (goal).

Unfortunately, authors, even researchers, often fail to identify all these elements of their phenomenon. But usually we can infer the items that fit in these pigeon holes if we have an article or a manuscript. Sometimes researchers who think they are studying spirituality fail to realize that they have forgotten their subject matter and slipped into related constructs in the other quadrants.

Let's take as additional practice in naming elements, with two very different philosophies of reality. We'll extract the major elements of each perspective. We might consider one of these sample philosophies to have major elements of spirituality and consider the other not to have such philosophies.

Sample Philosophy A: Life, including intelligent human life, is an event caused by the happen-chance collision of certain molecules with certain other molecules. The world is *out there*, separate from the perceiver. The extant world and human beings were not predetermined but evolved from matter, indeed, from a chance molecular event.

The way that healing takes place in this philosophy, involves investigating those molecular events and manipulating them so that the desired linkages take place and the undesired ones don't. Manipulating the elements to create the *right* collisions gives us control over results.

Here's how one might extract the four main elements from this theory:

Content—molecules
Process—accidental collision, interactions
Context—a world removed from the agent (observer/researcher)—a place where accidental events happen
Goal
    a. —in creating this world: none, happen-chance
    b. —in healing: whatever choices motivate the one manipulating the elements

Sample Philosophy B: Reality consists of God's ideas materializing in the form of a physical universe. Thought (or imagination) is the first step in manifesting anything, either by God or—to a lesser degree—by human beings. Thought forms stay alive by virtue of the intentionality put into them. Imagining plus intention creates form. Thought forms create reality and they stay alive by virtue of the energy put into them. A simple formula might be that the energy system plus consciousness equals manifestation of form.

The individual shares a holographic oneness with the universe. Humans are an inseparable part of the universe. Healing involves coming into mindfulness of our inseparable nature and using the patterns of imagination and intention.

Here's how one might extract the four main elements from this theory:

Content—mind (materializing ideas)
Process—intention and imagination
Context—the world of idea and creators (this world is not removed from the creator)
Goal
    a. —in creating this world: what the creator intends
    b. —in healing: what the human agent intends

Notice that both these philosophies address *matter* and *mind*. In this aspect, these philosophies are virtually at opposite ends of a continuum, with Philosophy A predominant in matter and Philosophy B predominant in mind. There could be, of course, other locations on the continuum, for example, a midpoint where mind and matter are indivisible. But we will continue with our illustrations at the opposite ends of the continuum. Not every philosophy has mind and matter as its important anchors, but they are convenient attachments when we're going to look at appropriate research methods. Notice that nursing, as well as concepts of spirituality, would be very different under these two notions of reality.

Now that we have an initial assessment of each philosophy as to content, process, context, and goal, we can ask about the appropriate research methods. How does a philosophy relate to a research question that supposedly asks a question about that described world?

Obviously, the question asked must be about some aspect of that world. Just as the philosophy has a process, so does the research. The processes of the philosophy and the research process must be compatible if the research is to mean anything. The main value to be achieved in matching a philosophy and a research method is *consistency*. In other words, the method of research must be capable of answering the question asked.

Recall that in Philosophy A, *content* is *molecules* (or pieces of matter). And there is an assumption that the world of matter exists out there, apart from the viewer/researcher of it. Often, philosophies aren't complete and here is a case in point. There is, however, an implied *method of thinking* that can be associated with Philosophy A: In this case, wholes are made up of their parts: molecules join with other molecules to create this envisioned world. This description starts at molecules; it could as easily have started at atoms. Clearly, one can assume (in the absence of other evidence) that molecules and their interactions kept up the collision process, making more and more complex forms. In this example, the parts comprise the whole. One explains this philosophy by reference to its parts. Therefore, the method of thinking in the philosophy (explaining the whole by its parts) should be repeated in the method of research for consistency. The philosophy has a method; so does the research.

If instead we have Philosophy B's defining reality, then we have radically different content: *thought (imagination)* and *intention*—not accidentally colliding molecules, but *intention* directed by a mind, an intellect (of God or man). And thought directs and maintains materialization which is simply an effect.

Philosophy A starts with matter; Philosophy B starts with mind in the form of thoughts. Hence, in B our method is not at all separate from the creator, God or man. The creator is very much part of the reality. Indeed thought and intention (factors in the creator) cause what comes into being.

Looking at the parts alone (the things that come into being) won't tell us much in this case because one must look higher in the system to see how it works. Unlike Philosophy A, knowing the parts in B doesn't tell us how the system works. In Philosophy B, we see that the parts are more than additive. They are explained by their participation in the whole (the mind of the creator).

Hence, research that fits A would be inconsistent for B—and vice versa. If we were to divide the world into just these two philosophies, we would have two very different ends of a continuum. They happen to be the two ends nursing has long used and about which it still argues. In Wilber's terms, Philosophy B deals with intentions (upper left-hand quadrant), while Philosophy A deals with molecules (upper right).

The appropriate method of thought for Philosophy A is termed *Logistic*. It will seem very familiar to nurses because of its use in the medical model. It is *reductionistic*, that is, it explains a thing by reference to its parts. Much of science works that way. For example, water is explained as two hydrogen atoms combined with one oxygen atom. The logistic system of thought is additive and moves downward in explaining. In our society, this form of explanation (and research) seems very natural. This is the model that has been so successful in molding modern medical research and much of modern nursing research.

One method fitting Philosophy B is labeled *Dialectic*. It explains things by reference to the larger entities in which they participate. In nursing, we often call our dialectic theories holistic, that is, they explain things in the opposite direction from a logistic method. Here one might explain water by saying that it participates in solving thirst, in renewing the planet, and so on, ultimately in the mind or intention of God. In nursing a therapy that affects the whole person, not just a part of him, often operates this way.

Holistic (dialectic) thought moves upward to explain things, and at the new level, unlike logistic thought, the result will be more than merely the sum of its parts: It will be different than its parts. In philosophy the combined new entity is often called the *Synthesis* to focus on the fact that it is different from its parts, known as the *Thesis* and the *Antithesis*.

Dialectic and logistic thought are two patterns, and they happen to fit our two examples here. There are also operational and problematic thought patterns.

Operational thought uses the method of making either/or discriminations. Medicine uses this system and calls it differential diagnosis. Either it's cancer or it's benign. If it's cancer, we can treat it by either resection or radiology, and so forth. Although the thought pattern is either/or, there may be more than just two options in any discrimination process. In computer programs, we call this branching logic, but the branching is always downward—making finer and finer differentiations. Modern computer programs often include branching techniques along with logistic systems.

Problematic thought will be familiar to nurses who once used the Weed system of charting or those who studied John Dewey's classic (1938). Problem identification and hypothesis testing is the focus here. Half the operations have to do with defining the problem accurately. Then the solutions *suggest themselves*, says Dewey. And one tests the most logical solution (an hypothesis) first, then the next, and so on until one finds the solution that works.

The focus of this method is on correct identification of the problem as much as on the hypothesis testing. For example, I was once called in on a consultation where the Nursing Vice President declared that her registered nurses and licensed practical nurses hated each other. She wanted me to interact with the staff using the popular psychology of the moment, which happened to be the method labeled *I'm okay; you're okay*. Obviously, her assumption was that it was a psychological problem.

But I first asked to look at her job descriptions for these staff roles, their assignments, and their pay scales. I found that they had radically different pay rates, yet their assignments were virtually identical. The Nursing Vice President had ignored the first part of problem solving: finding the correct problem. The underlying problem was economic, not psychological. And the wrong diagnosis inevitably leads to the wrong solution. Any amount of psychological intervention might have made a difference for a very short period of time, but then the original problem would have reemerged.

This, incidentally, is the chief problem that occurs when a consultant who is attached to a particular scheme is hired. One-size-fits-all solutions don't work when the problems are different.

In one sense, Logical Positivism suffered from this problem. It was a case of one-method-fits-all. And it simply wasn't true. One thing that encouraged nursing to stay overlong with Logical Positivism was that it talked the same language as medicine, in other words the medical model of thinking (Wilber's upper right-hand quadrant). Medicine didn't really get into alternative/complementary health practices (and possibly left quadrant thinking) until the Office of Alternative Medicine started giving funds for research in that model. One will recognize that the medical model (logistic or operational thought) is still dominant in nurse practitioner education. The clarity of answers on these models has appeal when the external viewpoint can be maintained.

Nursing programs of a holistic sort have developed as competition to nursing practitioner programs of the above type. They may be characterized by holistic principles or may be a mixed bag (for example, Dossey [1997] and Dossey, Keegan, & Guzzeta [2000]). Dossey speaks of being and doing. Her being principles (the nurse helps just by his/her presence) are holistic, but her doing principles (nursing actions) are often a mix of holistic and logistic. Although many of her principles are holistic, they don't preclude logistic elements—such as giving medications. In contrast, therapies like visualization and meditation are therapies that affect the whole person rather than aiming at his parts.

Now that we've discussed the methods of thought that could be used, let's get back to our two philosophies. Remember we are looking for consistency and compatibility between the thinking processes involved in the philosophy and the research method used to investigate it.

Research itself has many methods and we often reduce them to two main categories: qualitative and quantitative. You can almost separate these two types of research by the words they choose for their elements:

Qualitative	Quantitative
Mind	Brain
Consciousness	Beta brain waves

Not surprisingly, most people prefer to do one of these two types of research over the other. Quantitative people like to deal—so they often say—with the *real world*. What they usually mean is a world that can be known apart from the perceptions of the researcher. "Just let me count the cases, and I'll tell you which therapy works best."

Quantitative people like research derived from theories that look at the world from a removed, objective perspective. They like operationalized terms. They want to be able to tell whether something is X or Y with no ambiguity.

In quantitative approaches, there is a predictable world outside of the human researcher. When we do research, we learn the facts about that world. We all live in the same world, and the world responds to us in the same way. If vancomycin eliminates organism X, in one person, it will do that in another. Yes, there can be variables that influence outcomes, but they are identifiable—for example, the age and initial level of debilitation of the patient. One can work out percentages.

Hence, we can talk about outcomes of morbidity and mortality with predictability for groups. Goals can be identified in terms of desirable outcomes, usually the same for all persons with the same condition. Goals often deal with absence of disease or return to optimal function in activities of daily living.

If a patient does not share these goals, something is wrong with him or her, and he or she should be encouraged to conform with the predetermined desirable outcomes. Predetermined outcomes represent the end goals of action, and they often comprise the variables to be measured in quantitative research. Usually, people who prefer quantitative research are drawn to subject matters that fit that modality. But not always. The rash of quantitative studies supposedly on spirituality proves that point.

On the other hand, qualitative people like to deal with concepts, especially complex concepts that may be difficult to clarify. Subtle differences will intrigue them. Qualitative people like to fret over things and deal with subtle and subjective or intersubjective phenomena.

For the qualitative researcher, the individual's perception is the important thing to understand. To know/study the individual's thoughts, feelings, and interpretations is what matters. And this becomes important when we turn to the subject of spirituality because it is a state that is difficult, if not impossible, to identify as a quantitative variable. (The reader is reminded of Fowler's considerable work in trying to pin down levels of faith in Chapter 2.)

Even where one makes a scale or qualifying statements, like Fowler's statements (research using structuralism), there are still challenges in sorting the examples. I'm suggesting that when one researches spirituality with a quantitative tool, one has shifted from Wilber's left-hand quadrants to the right-hand quadrants. Spirituality is simply not a subject matter that can be separated from the one (or ones) experiencing it.

One common way that shift is made is to talk about religion instead of spirituality. Religions, of course, have spiritual values, but they also have variables that can be measured. After all, they are systems that have been codified, where certain beliefs have been accepted with certitude. And there are rituals, attendances, and other aspects that can be measured.

TYPES OF RESEARCH

For the reader who wants a sense of the difference between qualitative and quantitative research methods, here is a small list of research methods from each side.

Qualitative Methods

1. *Phenomenology* (upper left quadrant, singular)—involves looking within one person's perceptions. This concerns how it feels from within. It concerns experience of or about some object by virtue of its content or meaning. Sensory qualities of phenomena—perceptions, emotions, volition, and awareness—will be involved. This method seeks to find the meaning things have in the lived-world experience. It is the study of structures of experiences or consciousness from a first-person point of view.

2. *Hermeneutics* (lower left quadrant, plural)—the art and science of understanding and interpreting linguistic and nonlinguistic expressions. In trying to understand what people intend, the researcher looks at the hidden meanings in texts, histories, or recorded dialogs. Hermeneutics assumes that the literal meaning may mask deeper meanings, and the attempt is to reach those meanings. While phenomenology looks through *one person's eyes*, hermeneutics takes a broader view—through the eyes of a group or a society.

3. *Grounded Theory* (lower left quadrant, plural)—emphasizes generation of theory from data. It is a research method that operates almost in a reverse fashion to traditional research. Rather than beginning with a hypothesis, it begins by collecting data that seem to fit the concept (or theory) being explored.These data are then codified until the data collected no longer

reveal new categories. The categories then are used to create a theory. In essence, this research begins without a theory and strives to create one. One is immediately reminded of the direction of dialectic thought—upward from elements to the synthesis.

4. *Structuralism* (lower left quadrant, plural)—seeks patterns that connect phenomenological findings, posing questions to large numbers of people, seeing if their answers fall into categories. When this technique is effective, one often finds that categories may be differentiated by levels. We then derive theories like Maslow's, Piaget's, Erikson's, or Fowler's stages.

Quantitative Methods

1. *Classical Experimental Design* (upper right quadrant, singular)— compares control groups and treatment groups, and randomized clinical trials are typically used. Classical experimental design is based on manipulating the independent variable and measuring the effect on the dependent variable. Exploring the relationships between the variables obviously is a logistic thought method.

   The classical experimental method is a perfect match for right-hand quadrants. It compares effects of one variable to effects of another (or a lack of the variable). The method itself is reductionistic. And it is not influenced by the researcher. The assumption in this method is that the world is *out there*, and if various researchers carry out identical procedures, they will get identical results. The separation of the investigated world from the investigator is an important part of the method. It doesn't matter who is looking through the microscope (assuming they know how).

2. *Survey Lists, Census Data, and Demographics* (lower left quadrant, plural)—seek to record data on groups and make correlations when variables can't be manipulated. The important thing in creation of survey lists, census data, and demographics is to collect the most important data, eliminating nonessential data but keeping every bit of information that may be important in later correlations. This means that the researcher must know ahead of time what questions one wishes to answer when the data are collected.

MIXED CATEGORIES IN SPIRITUAL RESEARCH

Even when the method selected for research is clear, we face another problem: The subject matter of the research often demonstrates a mixing of religion and spirituality as if they were one. Although spirituality may (or may not) occur as a component of religion, religion is not a component of spirituality. The indiscriminate mixing of these two subjects makes any research under such a model meaningless. One can draw no meanings for spirituality or religion from such studies. Often, this confusion only shows up when one examines the separate categories or the questions in the measurement tool.

Alex Harris, Carl Thoresen, Michael McCullough, and David Larson (1999) note not only this problem but also another serious flaw: that studies of religion and spirituality often study the efficacy of therapeutic methods that may also be used without a religious/spiritual orientation. For example, meditation or a relaxation response can be used without either spirituality or religion being involved. So, here is another way that results can be confounded and attributed to religious/spiritual factors when there is no substantiation of the connection.

Although the studies examined by this evaluation group were published in 1999, newer studies show the same confusions. Further, many studies of spirituality/religion in health speak about *efficacy or effectiveness* without identifying just what they are efficacious in achieving or what they are effective in producing. When one reads on, searching for these unidentified variables, almost invariably they turn out to be health-related criteria, not spiritual/religious criteria. As we saw with Benson in Chapter 4, often measures of health are the hidden objectives of spiritual/religious treatments.

PSYCHO-SOCIO-NEURO-IMMUNOLOGY

An interesting phenomenon has occurred where upper right-hand investigators have tried to put together *all the pieces* involved in many medical investigations. What happens is that the number of pieces involved just keeps growing. As the title, psycho-socio-neuro-immunology indicates (or in some cases, psycho-socio-neuro-immuno-endocrinology), the number of systems involved in many medical therapies/inquiries has grown so extensive that they almost approach the place where every human system is involved in any condition and its treatment. The challenge in this thought, of course, is that saying *everything* is involved would mean a shift to the upper left-hand column.

Whereas many nurse practitioners focus on parts (diseases and conditions), holistic nurses deal with the person as a totality. This practice grew out of science also—a science that recognizes the multiple influences of each element on the human being as a whole. Originally, we heard of the science of psycho-sociobiology. Now we're up to psycho-socio-neuro-immunology (or longer) titles. Ironically, we now have a label that can be applied to both sides of the quadrant, but each treats the label in very different ways.

In keeping with Newtonian physics, the right quadrant assumes that a *real* world exists out there, separate from the researcher. Gary Zukav (2001) says:

> The old physics assumes that there is an external world which exists apart from us. It further assumes that we can observe, measure, and speculate about the external world without changing it. According to the old physics, the external world is indifferent to us and to our needs. (p. 31)

The new physics (we might say the left quadrant) in contrast, reveals a reality that can no longer be posed apart from the observer; as Zukav (2001) says:

> The new physics, quantum mechanics, tells us clearly that it is not possible to observe reality without changing it. If we observe a certain particle collision experiment, not only do we have no way of proving that the result would have been the same if we had not been watching it, all that we know indicates that it would not have been the same, because the result that we got was affected by the fact that we were looking for it. (p. 33)

Quantum mechanics recognizes the critical role the observer plays in creating the reality.

On the holistic side, the specific nurse *does* make a difference, even if he/she does exactly what another nurse does. And many therapies such as therapeutic touch, relaxation therapy, meditation, aroma therapy, massage, and visualization all affect the whole person, not just a part. Dossey (1997), for example, is heavily invested in alternate (or complementary) health care.

Most nurse practitioners and medics, however, are educated in the older model of an objective reality apart from the observer (the third-person objective position). This orientation assumes that only one sort of vision can give an accurate reflection on reality, and that orientation is the same for everyone.

Although this viewpoint is wrong at extreme ends of reality, it is still useful for many mid-range phenomena. Newtonian physics (and the world it sees) is a useful lie. Medical research, of course, falls happily in this middle range.

SUMMARY

To return to our original assertion, it appears that much research dealing with spirituality is invalid because it asks research questions that are inappropriate to questions of spirituality (a category mistake). Often variables from other quadrants of Wilber's Kosmos, for example, are substituted for questions that actually concern the concept of spirituality (from the upper left-hand quadrant).

Nurses, in particular, have been encouraged to keep their research in Wilber's upper right-hand quadrant (classical hypothesis testing), and this may lead them to pick topics that are only tangentially related to spirituality while believing they are investigating this subject matter. Sometimes, this shift involves substituting *religiosity* for *spirituality* because the form is more likely to have quantifiable variables.

Even where the true subject is religion, not every aspect of religion can be quantified. Religion is not a simple variable because it has both external aspects (like rituals and attendance) and internal values (like its spiritual values).

Yet, as we have discussed, even where a tool proclaims that it measures spirituality, it is possible that items in the tool may actually be about religion, not spirituality. Every tool must be examined for this flaw. Often tools mix religious and spiritual values. One cannot accept tools at face value.

Nevertheless, we have some substantive tools at our disposal, such as Fowler's Stages of Faith. The subject matter of spirituality lends itself to good research when it is placed in the proper context, most likely in Wilber's upper left quadrant.

REFERENCE

Zukav, G. (2001). *The dancing Wu Li masters: An overview of the new physics.* New York: Harper Collins Publishers (Perennial Classics).

BIBLIOGRAPHY

Dewey, J. (1938). *Logic: The theory of inquiry.* New York: Henry Holt and Company.
Dossey, B. M. (1997). *Core Curriculum for holistic nursing.* Gaithersburg, MD: Aspen Publishers.
Dossey, B. M., Keegan, K. L., & Guzzeta, C. E. (2000). *Holistic nursing: A handbook for practice* (3rd ed.). Gaithersburg, MD: Aspen Publishers.
Harris, A., Thoresen, C., McCullough, M., & Larson, D. (1999). Spirituality and religiously oriented health interventions. *Journal of Health Psychology, 4*(3), 413–433.
Wilber, K. (1996). *A brief history of everything.* Boston: Shambhala.
Wilber, K. (2007). *Integral spirituality.* Boston: Integral Books.

CHAPTER 6

Spirituality and Nursing Theory: A Miss or a Match?

Why do we keep putting spirituality in nursing theories? Is it because of our early heritage in both the arts and sciences? Is it time we turn that function over to the religious/spiritual experts? What do we have to lose, what to gain, by retaining spirituality in our nursing theories?

There are several *grand theories* of nursing, as well as a few *middle-range theories*, in which spiritual components are given high priority. If we look back at the problems already discussed (particularly in Chapters 2 and 5), we must ask how the choice to include spirituality as a major theme in a nursing theory can be both justified and enacted.

This doesn't mean that it's impossible to include spirituality as a major component of nursing; it just means that the theorist has a challenging job in creating the theory and making it work. How can elements from another discipline assume major importance in a theory designed to direct nursing care? How is this justified, and how is it played out?

In this chapter, we'll examine three theories with spiritual components: Barbara Dossey's *Theory of Integral Nursing*, Margaret Newman's *Theory of Health as Expanding Consciousness*, and Mary Elizabeth O'Brien's *Theory of Spiritual Well-Being in Illness*. The first two are grand theories, the last one is middle range.

There are additional theories of nursing with spiritual elements (e.g., Travelbee, 1971, and Watson, 2000), but I've selected these three because together they illustrate important points about inserting spirituality in nursing theories.

To a great degree, grand theories that were popular in the 70s and 80s have passed into nursing's history. Many grand theories with spiritual components seem less applicable today than in the past. Yet that isn't true for all the grand theories. For example, the theories of Barbara Dossey and colleagues have thrived for years in directing holistic programs of nursing. I suspect that Dossey's new theory (discussed here) will also be applied in holistic program of nursing, although it could be applied in any program of care.

Two important points must be made before we look at our theories individually. The first is that some readers may be puzzled as to why one or two of these theories are labeled as spiritual. Those readers who closely associate spirituality with religion may require a shift in focus. But those readers must remember our prior definition of spirituality: that spirituality refers to what is most meaningful, direction giving and purpose providing for the theorist. Spirituality is connectedness to the sacred, however that is conceived. Spirituality is also internal, affective, spontaneous, and private. With each illustration, we will examine what elements serve that spiritual function in the theory. O'Brien's theory, in contrast to the work of Dossey and Newman will sound more traditional with its mixed spiritual and religious elements.

Next we need to know that there are two different kinds of theories: *regular* theories complete with all their components, and *metatheories*. The metatheory, in contrast to the regular theory, is best envisioned as an empty structure into which the theory pieces may be placed. I like to think of a metatheory as a pigeonholed desk with many openings to hold the various contents. *Commonplace* is another term for a pigeonhole. A metatheory doesn't tell you what is *in* each pigeonhole; instead it tells you what pigeonholes exist and must be filled if you are to have a complete theory.

In other words, a metatheory is on a higher level. It is like the framework that will support the house, but until you know more, you might not know if a section will hold a family room or a bedroom. A metatheory defines the structure that will hold together the pieces of a subsequent theory. In fact, for many such structures, it might be possible to fill the slots with different content, making different theories that share the same pigeonholes (structure).

One can easily tell the difference between these two types of theories because the regular type has, so to speak, all the pieces, at least all the pieces the author has supplied. When you've finished reading this kind of theory, you could go out and apply it to patient care.

THEORY OF INTEGRAL NURSING

Dossey's new theory (in Dossey and Keegan, 2009) theory begins with a metatheory. (I should mention, when referring to a theory, if I call something the *first part*, I don't mean that this is when the author discusses it. I simply mean to indicate its location in the logical explication of a theory.)

Hence, Dossey begins with a metatheory, and this is my chief reason for selecting this theory. Indeed, few theorists create a metatheory when devising a theory. This effort means that Dossey has a strong commitment to this particular structure and these particular commonplaces. One of her chief commitments is to Ken Wilber's (1996, 2000) *Four Corners of the Kosmos*, his quadrants as we discussed in Chapter 5. The reader is referred back to that chapter to refresh his memory of this structure. (See Exhibits 5.1 and 5.2.)

Dossey combines Wilber's four-quadrant structure with some other structures that have had a long shelf life in nursing, for example, the commonplaces composed of nurse, person, health, and environment, Carper's (1978) so-called metaparadigm of nursing.

Here is a good place to get a feel for what a metatheory does. For any commonplaces in a set, we can ask the pertinent questions. In this case, those would be: Who or what comprises a nurse? Who or what comprises a person? What comprises health? And what is the environment in which this theory takes place?

As you can see, these commonplaces may look like terms that speak for themselves, but they are not. For example, later when we look at Newman's theory, we will see that *health* is defined as continuous expanding of one's consciousness. Granted, this isn't how one usually thinks of health, but for Newman's theory, that is what goes into the pigeonhole of health. And so it is with all the other empty slots. Each theory fills these commonplaces with its own unique components.

The same is true for Wilber's four quadrants. Any phenomenon selected will look different from these four perspectives. The reader may recall that the term, *mind*, in Wilber's upper left (*me*) quadrant was changed to the term *brain*, when in the upper right-hand (*it*) quadrant. Hence, these quadrants are also commonplaces.

Wilber has tended throughout his career, to continuously expand his system to where it becomes encyclopedic. It is not surprising that one of his books is titled *A brief history or everything* (1996). Dossey shows this same tendency to include many structures. Hence, she also adds Carper's patterns of knowing: personal, aesthetic, empiric, ethical, and sociopolitical knowing (added from White, 1995) and not knowing (added from Munhall, 1993). Notice again, we can ask, what is aesthetic knowledge in this theory? What is the system of ethics in this theory? In other words, we have commonplaces again.

Dossey builds her metatheory layer upon layer until all her commonplaces are combined around a central point. If you read Dossey's theory in its totality, you will see there is yet another structure in the metaparadigm, also borrowed from Wilber (2007), and named *all quadrants, all levels, all lines, all states, all types (AQAL)*. This again reflects Wilber's desire to be comprehensive, encyclopedic in his structuring of all reality. One challenge Dossey faces in adding this additional schema is that each of these additional factors (levels, lines, states, and types) will require definition. And they also have many subordinate variables within these categories, seven or eight being typical. The overall effect is to add an extensive number of additional variables to Dossey's metaparadigm.

By using two of Wilber's structures, Dossey is vulnerable to the same problem of having a tremendous number of items in her metaparadigm. Indeed, some nurses may complain that this level of comprehensiveness is more than what they want in their role. Also, most nurses would need some additional education in all these metatheory structures before being ready to move on to the other aspects of this total model.

One future complication in developing this metatheory is that these various structures (commonplaces) may also impact on each other. For example, it is possible that Carper's items, nurse, person, health, and environment, might change as they pass through Wilber's different quadrants.

Incidentally, one way you can tell that this portion of the theory is a metatheory is that you could go into the clinical area after learning this part of Dossey's model and still not know what to do for a patient. That's because the next step is filling these commonplaces (pigeonholes) with specific content.

Dossey adds one element from her *regular* theory to the metatheory: her primary element, *healing*. This element appears in the middle of the metatheory diagram connecting all these structures like a central pin holding a pinwheel together. However, because *healing* bridges everything, one particularly needs to ask if its definition can remain unchanged as it moves from one of Wilber's quadrants to the next. (Recall that *mind* shifted to *brain* in one quadrant change.) So we must ask if healing undergoes any similar changes in its definition.

Remember this is the first presentation of this theory and we must consider it a work in progress. Having completed her metatheory, Dossey moves on to identify and define variables in what I'm calling her *regular* theory. Interestingly, Dossey described more variables that would fall into Wilber's left-hand quadrants than those that would be placed in the right-hand quadrants. She justified this by specifying that other theories often leave out left-hand variables. So she sees this as compensation.

And we find the spirituality elements in this theory (the *regular* theory), in the left-hand quadrants. Her definition of spirituality is much like that we've used in this book, and she presents it as a transpersonal element under the lower left quadrant (which readers will remember is the *we* quadrant). In relation to the transpersonal element, Dossey says in Dossey and Keegan (2009):

. . . recognize the role of *spirituality* that is the search for the sacred or holy that involves feeling, thoughts, experiences, rituals, meaning, value, direction, and purpose. . . . (p. 34)

In addition, spirituality is also discussed under the *context* of the theory:

Spiritual meaning is related to how one deepens personal experience of a connection with the Divine. . . . (p. 31)

Dossey also adds structures of *content*, *context*, and *process* to her metatheory. Under the process element, she adds concepts of suffering, moral suffering, moral distress, and soul pain. Other elements of this theory often associated with spirituality—mindfulness, meditation, centering prayer, and conscious dying—all are presented under the upper left-hand quadrant (the *me* location).

Nor can we ignore the fact that healing, the central concept in this theory, is worded in a way that is highly compatible with spirituality. Healing is:

. . . the innate natural phenomenon that comes from within a person and describes the indivisible wholeness, the interconnectedness of all people, and all things. (p. 17)

Dossey gives us a good example of a theory that includes spirituality as one of its values. Dossey claims that this theory includes all of reality and that, of course, is its vulnerability. One must ask if that is too much to ask of the nurse. Dossey recognizes this weakness and says that the nurse will improve to the degree that he or she masters this content, thus recognizing that full understanding and application of her model is an ideal:

. . . to be integrally informed does not mean that we have to master all these areas; we just need to be aware of them and chose to integrate integral awareness and integral practice. (p. 29)

Summarizing Dossey's theory is complicated because it involves both a metatheory and an evolving *regular* theory of specifics. So far, we have barely mentioned the main vocabulary of the metatheory, which has to do with her title, *integral nursing*. The use of this term, integral, is also taken from Wilber, and Dossey differentiates it from her old commitment to holistic nursing, which she says is included but transcended (Wilber's way of dealing with subordinate phenomena in his theory work). Dossey defines an integral process as:

. . . a comprehensive way to organize multiple phenomenon of human experience and reality from four perspectives. . . . (p. 17)

Of her metatheory structures, Wilber's four Corners of the Kosmos is the model most discussed.

Yet we will need to focus on the *regular* theory to bring our analysis down to the arena of actual nursing care. At this level, one could summarize Dossey's theory by saying that *healing* is the nurse's (and the patient's) *goal*. And healing is described as, "the innate natural phenomenon within a person and describes the indivisible wholeness, the interconnectedness of all people, and all things" (p. 17). The *context* in which healing takes place is the whole of reality (as structured through the metatheory). Because this context of reality includes *everything*, then spirituality is a part of it.

The methods (process elements) that the nurse uses to help the patient achieve health are multifold, but one can extract aspects such as understanding one's own interior (the nurse working on self-understanding), presence, being with the patient, knowing, doing, mindfulness, deep listening, compassion, intention, and intuition, among others. By Dossey's definition of nursing actions in all four quadrants, we are faced with a plethora of processes.

The *content* of this theory, according to Dossey, is health and the elements of the metatheory structures. I would, of course, bring content down to the level beneath the metatheory and define it as the elements within that developing schema (the things in the pigeonholes). In this theory, they are multiple, with each element of the metatheory leading to more content items. Perhaps the simplest way to begin to define all these content items is to note that health is both *content* and *goal*. I'm grateful to Dossey for having included her metatheory in her theory presentation. It represents a major amount of work that not every theorist does.

THEORY OF HEALTH
AS EXPANDING CONSCIOUSNESS

Margaret Newman (2000) gives us a *regular* grand theory, that is, it does not contain a metatheory. That makes it simpler to interpret; we only need to deal with one theory level. In Dossey's model, spirituality was only one part. Newman's theory is more fully based in spirituality. Yet the form of spirituality may be difficult for some to recognize.

If *healing* is Dossey's main theme, then *evolving consciousness* is Newman's theme. Indeed, it is the *goal* of this theory. Life is about one's level of consciousness becoming more and more complex. And it is the nurse's goal to help patients "recognize the power that is within them to move to higher levels of consciousness" (p. xv). She states:

> From the moment we are conceived to the moment we die, in spite of changes that accompany aging, we manifest a pattern that identifies us as a particular person. (p. 71)

For Newman, that pattern gets defined in two ways, (1) as an energy field and (2) as a progression of psychological events that create a recognizable pattern of behavior and being. The most significant events of a lifetime reveal the pattern. Yet interruptions in pattern, even chaos, are important because these moments allow for revisions to a higher complexity. Pattern is described this way:

> . . . life is evolving in the direction of higher levels of consciousness . . . a fluctuating field that periodically transcends itself and shifts into a higher order of functioning. . . . (p. 43)

Even what we normally label as disease may serve a function, namely causing a disruption in pattern that may be solved by shifting to a higher and more complex level of consciousness. Hence, disease and wellness can both contribute to the human goal of evolving into ever-increasing complexity, that is, balance, imbalance, then balance again:

> We evolve by having our own equilibrium thrown off balance and then discovering how to attain a new state of balance, temporarily, and then moving on to another phase of disequilibrium. (p. 21)

> The pattern being signaled by disease (as well as non-disease) can be seen and understood in terms of a pattern of energy. (p. 17)

I have always wondered how Newman still recognizes a person's pattern if that pattern is continuously evolving. Is there ever so much change that the original pattern has evolved beyond recognition? This is a question Newman doesn't answer.

Because this evolving is one's greatest goal in life, it meets the criterion for being the most meaningful and therefore the most spiritual task of living. And this is how Newman's theory enters the domain of spirituality. It's all about spirituality, and spirituality *is* evolving consciousness. Hence, Newman identifies evolving consciousness as the most important spiritual state. Evolving consciousness is both health and a life's goal:

> The process of the evolution of consciousness is the process of health. (p. 43)

Although she does not recommend actual energy measurement (an interesting omission), she does see the nurse identifying the psychological, emotional, and interpretive patterns of the patient's lifetime. This expands with time and experience to also incorporate common patterns of various diseases. This analysis could be called the first *process* of nursing: finding a patient's pattern and checking it out with the patient to see if it has been correctly interpreted.

The nurse assists the patient in returning to the path of evolving consciousness by helping him or her readjust his or her pattern of development when it has slipped into chaos. Newman (2000) defines the process in this way in reference to groups of patients:

> . . . presentations of the evolving pattern of each of the participants' lives is to help them to gain insight into their pattern and reveal the action potential of the pattern. (p. 91)

Newman calls this *presentational construing.* She describes it as a hermeneutic, dialectic approach that "seeks to capture the evolving, transformative nature of the nurse–client relationship" (p. 87).

> The responsibility of the nurse is not to make people well, or to prevent them getting sick, but to assist people to recognize the power that is within them to move to higher levels of consciousness. (p. xv)

> The task is not to try to change another person's pattern but to recognize it as information that depicts the whole and relate to it as it unfolds. (p. 13)

The second element of *process* is helping the patient repattern if he desires to do so:

> Each of us at some time in our lives is brought to a point when the "old rules" do not work anymore . . . *the crux of life* is to learn the new rules. (p. 99)

In essence, the nurse assists the patient in learning the new rules.

Newman makes a point of decimating the sort of thinking (reductive) that explains things by reference to their parts (Wilber's upper right-hand quadrant):

> The traditional scientific paradigm calls for predictable outcomes in situations, outcomes that have the potential to "fix" problems. The new paradigm calls for action evolving out of pattern recognition. (p. 52)

> To intervene with a particular result in mind is to say we know what form the pattern of expanding consciousness will take, and we don't. (p. 97)

Newman would find the fixation on outcome objectives of today's accrediting bodies totally antithetical to her notion of nursing. The *context* in which her nursing takes place is a world of energy and ideas, a world that itself is evolving and changing.

Just as Dossey's concept of health is both the main *content* and the main *goal* of her theory, so it is with Newman's principle of evolving conscious. It also is *content* and *goal* at the same time.

Newman's definition of the human being is also unique:

> . . . the human being is unitary, that is, cannot be divided into parts, and is inseparable from the larger unitary field. (p. xviii)

The human being is mind and energy first, and he or she is coextensive with all of reality. Respecting the nature of the human being, the nurse doesn't attempt to fix or change him or her. He or she is a recognizable component, an energy signature, but he or she is still a part of a larger whole. In all its elements, Newman's theory is dialectic (explaining thoughts by reference to the larger wholes in which they participate). It is never reductive and never explains a thing by isolating its parts.

I selected Newman's theory for my second illustration because it is based around a spiritual theme (evolving consciousness). Second, and most importantly, it illustrates that spirituality is based on the aspect that gives the most meaning to one's life, the phenomenon that most reaches the Divine for this theorist. It need not be a theme that we are used to thinking of as spiritual.

THEORY OF SPIRITUAL WELL-BEING IN ILLNESS

Mary Elizabeth O'Brien's (2008) theory gives us two more theory values: (1) a middle-range presentation and (2) a more traditional interpretation of the human being and of spiritual values. At times, she calls the human being one with needs of body, mind, and spirit (p. 87), and at other times a physical, psychosocial, and spiritual being. (p. 89) In either case, these are relatively traditional interpretations.

With O'Brien's theory, we are dealing with a mix of religious and spiritual variables that probably could not be fully separated for research purposes. If we had to label this theory, we would be safer labeling it *religious* rather than *spiritual*. After all, we know that religion may have a spiritual component, but spirituality does not inherently have a religious component. And many of O'Brien's content terms have specific religious meanings.

Middle-range theories are the most promulgated at the moment, and O'Brien's *Theory of Spiritual Well-Being in Illness* fits that category. O'Brien has done much research and publishing on this theory.

For all three illustrative theories, I would have liked to contain my analysis to the author's chapter on theory. For Dossey and O'Brien I was able to do that. But for Newman, I had to include elements from all over her book because her theory is distributed throughout. For O'Brien's work, then, I was able to contain discussion to her theory chapter, recognizing that some of her definitions were in the other chapters. Her use of this theory in research also affected how she defines her components.

Although this theory appears in a nursing text and is discussed in relation to nursing care, the theory itself is not exactly a nursing theory. Its components (p. 90) could just as easily be used by ministers, priests, and other religions workers or by physicians and other health care workers. Note that we could have said the same about Newman's theory. Expanding consciousness certainly is not a principle limited to nursing.

O'Brien is correct that her theory is middle range because it is limited by its focus on spiritual well-being and by its focus on illness. The theory does not purport to address spiritual well-being in every aspect of life. Nor does it purport to discuss spiritual well-being in health. In this regard, it is neither like Dossey's theory (whose content was all of reality) nor like Newman's theory, where expanding consciousness is a principle driving all of life, not just illness.

In brief, O'Brien's theory contains six subordinate categories that comprise most of the *content* of her theory:

1. Personal faith
2. Spiritual contentment
3. Religious practice
4. Severity of illness
5. Social support
6. Stressful life events

These *content* components would appear to be rather evenly distributed between spiritual/religious variables (1–3) and illness-related variables (4–6). However, that initial judgment is challenged because the nonreligious variables have only one to three subset categories in each, whereas the spiritual/religious categories have five or six subsets each. If one were to total up all these subset components, spiritual/religious variables would weigh much heavier than the illness-related variables. And it gives us a clue as to where O'Brien's real interest lies.

Briefly, the subsets for the six variables follow:

1. *Personal faith*: belief in God's existence, peace in spiritual beliefs, confidence in God's power, strength from faith beliefs, and trust in God's providence.
2. *Spiritual contentment*: satisfaction with faith, feeling of closeness to God, lack of fear, reconciliation, security in God's love, and faithfulness.
3. *Religious practice*: support of a faith community, affirmation in worship, encouragement of spiritual companions, consolation from prayer, and communication with God through religious practices.
4. *Severity of illness*: degree of functional impairment.
5. *Social support*: family, friends, and caregivers.
6. *Stressful life events*: emotional, sociocultural, and financial.

The definitions of all these terms are elsewhere in this book. Suffice it to say they are operationalized for purposes of research. The reader will note, however, that many of these terms are religious. Indeed, some of them are given a *religious* interpretation rather than their meaning in the common vernacular. For example, *God's providence, reconciliation,* and *consolation from prayer* have religious interpretations.

Given the total number of subsets, O'Brien's theory has far more *content* components than Newman's theory but fewer components than Dossey's. It is clear that these many elaborations have been created by O'Brien in designing tools for research. However, one labels these variables and their subsets, these plus the other main theory components, come up to 31 items. Both O'Brien and Dossey bear the vulnerability of having far too many variables for the nurse to retain in his or her mind while providing care.

All six of the major components listed above spill into what must be assumed to be a final decision point labeled *Finding spiritual meaning in the experience of illness.* In O'Brien's visual model (p. 90), directional arrows from these six items all lead to this summative item. Then, without further intervention, this summative judgment leads directly to the final theory component: *Spiritual well-being in illness.*

Because there are no other elements between these two items, one must assume that these two components correlate directly. This direct association leads us to ask: Is *Finding spiritual meaning in the experience of illness* the only variable that determines *spiritual well-being in illness?* Apparently, O'Brien closely associates *finding spiritual meaning* with *spiritual well-being.* Indeed, she says:

> . . . an ill individual is presented as having the ability to find spiritual meaning in the experience of illness, which can ultimately lead to an outcome of spiritual well-being. . . . (p. 89)

Are there no other unnamed variables that contribute to these correlations? More important, could we make a case that the association of *finding spiritual meaning in the experience of illness* with *spiritual well-being* is not inevitable? I think, for example, of a very religious woman who thoroughly viewed illnesses and injuries as accidental instead of associating them with divine meaning. When her son was killed, for example, she said to me about life: "It's a turkey shoot." She found no spiritual meaning in illness or injury, yet she had a high sense of spiritual well-being despite the many episodes in her life that might relate to the *turkey shoot* principle.

When I find such an assumption of correlation like the one O'Brien makes here, I immediately wonder if we may have an issue of context. Is finding spiritual meaning in illness necessarily a prerequisite for spiritual well-being? Or is it possible to separate these variables?

My objection is that the theory may be set in a hidden context, and it might not work so well if subjects varied. Let's imagine a hypothetical example. We have before us two patients, both of whom believe in God. But the Gods they believe in are very different. Patient A believes in a God much like the one assumed in this model, one who made and loves man, who as the creator, is separate from man, his creation. (Notice this would be the *context* of this Theory A.)

Patient B, on the other hand, believes that God is everything, a principle that distributed itself in the Big Bang. Hence, everything, including Patient B himself, is a part of God. Man is not separate from God; he is a small component of God. Here the *context* is quite different from that in Theory A. Because most people have Version A of God (that one Patient B irreverently calls *Big Daddy in the Sky*), he or she has been unable to find a faith community in which he or she feels comfortable. (One can imagine what this does to his or her scores on the religious subsets of this theory.)

So Patient B doesn't join a church, although ironically, he or she is much more spiritual than Patient A who belongs to and attends regularly, a faith community. Patient B, unlike Patient A, has earned his or her spiritual spurs the hard way—years of intensive thought and study on the subject and intensive personal experiences that confirm for him or her, his or her perception of God. This different viewpoint (and his scoring on the mixed spiritual/religious items in this theory) will probably give the researcher a summation that is a very false reading for Patient B.

In essence, O'Brien's theory and the associated research scales will probably work very well for large groups of people who hold traditional notions of God: people who belong to traditional Judeo-Christian religions. But the model simply won't fit everyone.

Few models do fit all, but the exceptions one can imagine lay this model open to question. On the other hand, we could not ask such questions of Dossey or Newman because their grand theories did not generate direct research questions. Further, if O'Brien specifies that her research subjects must be from Judeo-Christian faiths, then her research would avoid the *context* issue I described above.

One additional comment about O'Brien's discussion of her diagram: Many of her comments describe testing between *quality of life* and the variables in her model. Many variables of quality of life are mentioned (e.g., *hope for the future, being positive about life, being able to get through difficulties, feeling loved, and life satisfaction*), yet no relation between quality of life and the theory components are made in the diagram. It would be useful if this apparently important variable were included in the theory diagram.

Still, one must say that openness to research is one of the advantages of a middle-range theory: it is more accessible for testing.

Note also that, as we will discuss more fully in Chapter 9, it is impossible to separate spirituality and research in this theory. Because many of O'Brien's variables include religion-specific items (e.g., many subsets under *Religious Practice*), one would have to call this theory religious rather than spiritual. (Remember from Chapter 1 that religion may have a spiritual component, but spirituality need not have a religious component.) My point is that the *context* in this theory may be unrecognized by the author.

Next we need to isolate the *goal* of this theory and that is easy: *spiritual well-being in illness*. The *process* (what methods the nurses uses) includes:

. . . assess and evaluate their patients' spiritual needs and, if warranted, to institute appropriate spiritual care interventions. (p. 87)

These spiritual care interventions turn out to be the following:

. . . nurses facilitate either the enhancement of, or in some cases the return to, religious practices that may have waned or even been abandoned by a patient. . . . (p. 92)

. . . a nurse may be able to serve as a referral agent assisting sick persons in finding some relief for a functional impairment. (p. 92)

A nurse may also serve as a "bridge" facilitating communication with family and friends if these relationships have become strained due to illness or disability. (p. 92)

. . . the nurse may have the opportunity to guide, advise, teach, or support an ill patient in regard to a variety of emotional, sociocultural, and even financial concerns. . . . (pp. 92–93)

It would appear that many of these interventions (except the first one) lend themselves to psychological interpretations as easily as religious ones. (This is just an observation, not a criticism.) Yet she clearly states a religious *purpose*:

> It is for the purpose of identifying, supporting, and strengthening the influence of these spiritual resources, in relation to sickness or disability, that the nursing theory of spiritual well-being in illness has been developed. (p. 89)

The first intervention (which might include returning the patient to religious practices that have waned) would be vulnerable to the challenge of possibly stopping the patient in his journey toward a higher level of spiritual faith (see Chapter 1). Yet one must say this is in keeping with the theory's goal, that is, *spiritual well-being in illness*.

Recall that in Chapter 4, spirituality is often dismissed in its own right and seen merely as a tool to reach health goals. One reason I picked O'Brien's theory is that she has a spiritual goal as well as a health goal, and she is consistent in that pursuit. Because this is a middle-range theory, she doesn't face the criticism that Newman might receive—that her theory makes her form of spirituality all of nursing and all of reality. O'Brien can simply answer that this theory was never meant to explain all of nursing.

As indicated earlier, this theory could also be used by a religious professional after obtaining the original assessment on the health elements from a health care professional. Indeed, the minister or priest might be more competent than the nurse in assessing the religious/spiritual components of the theory.

I selected O'Brien's theory to show both the advantages and vulnerabilities of a middle-range theory. The advantage is that the theory can be researched; the disadvantage is that the research can be closely inspected to see if it truly measures the theory elements. Another reason I chose this theory is that it comes closer to most people's traditional beliefs concerning spirituality/religion.

OTHER ASPECTS OF SPIRITUAL/RELIGIOUS NURSING THEORIES

I'll only mention two other theoretical challenges for nursing theory—first, nursing's affinity for value commitments, and next, the challenge of deciding what comes first: nursing or spiritual values.

Nursing's Affinity for Values

Unlike many other professions, nursing doesn't start with what is given. No one says what chemistry *should* achieve before they figure out how it works. Yes, we add a science element but that comes after we've set our values. Unlike the hard sciences that start with the givens, we start with what we want to achieve for the patient. Nowhere is that more evident than in today's nursing practice where so many of our processes begin with the setting of objectives. For a long time, we have used such things as care maps and case norms to determine our goals for any given group of patients.

Usually, care goals are the same for every patient with the same disease or the same loss of function. Most fields have a very good idea of their boundaries before they determine what they will attempt. Yet we often overestimate what spiritual goals can be achieved by the nurse. Spirituality pushes our boundaries.

Not all nursing theories have a spiritual component. But virtually all nursing theories have a *value* component in that they are proposals for how nursing *ought* to be organized rather than being grounded in research observations of what actually happens.

What Comes First: Nursing Values or Spiritual Values?

When another discipline is heavily involved in a nursing theory, there is always a question of whether a theory can serve two masters. If not, which element has the most significance? One solution is to wed the two disciplines so that the nursing element *is* the spiritual element. We saw this tactic taken in Newman's theory. Another tactic (one we saw with O'Brien) is to limit the theory to middle range so that only one aspect of nursing is vulnerable to being taken over by the secondary discipline. In Dossey's case, we have yet another approach, namely the spiritual element is just one content element among many others.

Although one can argue that spirituality is an extraneous element in a nursing theory, the countervailing argument is that, like it or not, nurses are forced to deal with patients' spiritual dilemmas. So *de facto*, spirituality becomes a part of nursing. There is no easy answer between these two positions.

SUMMARY

This chapter started by asking if spirituality was a match or mismatch for nursing theory. Clearly, we have some nurse theorists who have been able to integrate spirituality into their theories. We might even say there is a certain trend to go back and reattach the element of spirituality to the definition of the human being: body, mind, and spirit as it was so many years ago.

At least our holistic nursing theories claim we must nurse the whole, indivisible human being. So perhaps we can justify spirituality as part of our theory constructions. If this is true, however, perhaps we need to better consider how to prepare nurses for spiritual tasks and how to manage both nursing objectives and spiritual objectives when they compete with each other. Can spirituality find a place in nursing theory? Yes, but it will take delicate handling to resolve the issues that arise when this is done.

REFERENCES

Dossey, B., & Keegan, L. (2009). *Holistic nursing: A handbook for practice* (5th ed., pp. 17–46). Sudbury, MA: Jones and Bartlett.

Newman, M. (2000). *Health as expanding consciousness* (2nd ed.). Sudbury, MA: Jones and Bartlett.

O'Brien, M. E. (2008). *Spirituality in nursing: Standing on holy ground* (3rd ed., pp. 85–94). Sudbury, MA: Jones and Bartlett.

BIBLIOGRAPHY

Carper, B. A. (1978). Fundamental patterns of knowing in nursing. *Advances in Nursing Science, 1*(1), 13–23.

Munhall, P. L. (1993). Unknowing: Toward another pattern of knowing in nursing. *Nursing Outlook, 41*(3), 125–128.

Travelbee, J. (1971). *Interpersonal aspects of nursing*. Philadelphia: F. A. Davis.

Watson, J. (2000). *Toward a caring curriculum: New pedagogy for nursing*. Sudbury, MA: Jones and Bartlett.

Watson, J. (2008). *Nursing: The philosophy and science of caring* (Rev. ed.). Boulder, CA: University Press of Colorado.

White, J. (1995). Patterns of knowing: Review, critique, and update. *Advances in Nursing, Science, 17*(2), 73–86.

Wilber, K. (1996). *A brief history of everything*. Boston: Shambhala.

Wilber, K. (2000). *Integral psychology*. Boston: Shambhala.

Wilber, K. (2007). *Integral spirituality*. Boston: Integral Books.

CHAPTER 7

Should Spiritual Care Be Taught in Nursing Education?

Is spiritual care a legitimate nursing function? Is it logical to expect nursing education to incorporate aspects of spirituality? If so, what are the challenges? In Chapter 2, we recognized that there are many levels of spiritual development. How can we educate nursing students who may themselves be at different levels of spiritual development?

Then there is the necessity of separating spirituality from religion as we saw in Chapter 1, especially when our students come from many different religions. However, it may be easier said than done for many potential teachers.

Additionally, we realized that we cannot teach spirituality merely as content. That simply is not adequate. It must be inculcated into the nurse as well if he or she is to draw on it in practice. Spirituality involves one's deepest values not just cognitive content. How do we handle a subject matter that requires inculcation as well as traditional teaching? What content allows us to inculcate in our students notions of spirituality?

IS SPIRITUAL CARE MISPLACED IN NURSING EDUCATION?

In the distant past, it was assumed that spiritual care was intrinsic to the nursing role. Indeed, if one goes back far enough (let's say medieval times), spiritual care may have been the only thing, other than comfort measures, that could be offered to most patients. When nursing was in its infancy as a profession or occupation, nurses were taught to care for the body, mind, and spirit. It was assumed that the nurse was capable of doing so. However, it was highly likely that the nurse and patient shared at least a similar religious orientation and possibly a similar spiritual heritage. The world then seldom presented nurses with patients from diverse cultures. On the whole, it was a world of more insular societies. Multicultural care was a thing of the future.

Further, the original notion of spirituality often served as the stimulus to recruit nurses with a different sort of dedication to nursing. Nursing was seen as a religious or spiritual lifestyle choice, that is, the choice that dominated and controlled one's whole life. That ideology of nursing has changed over the years, and the content of nursing curricula has also changed. Nursing moved to caring for the bio-psycho-social man. This change eliminated the spiritual element or converted it into psychology, sociology, or both. This trend accelerated in the late 50s and early 60s as nursing moved toward asserting itself as a science. Even the original descriptions of nursing as an art and a science shifted, and the profession began to be described more exclusively as a science.

Part of this was in response to other professions resisting nursing's move toward professionalization. Yes—primarily physicians—but other disciplines as well. Nursing was seen as not fitting the academic mold. It is no wonder that nursing worked to hide those aspects of care that would stand out as art rather than science. Making all traces of spirituality part of psychology was one way to achieve that end. Indeed, nursing worked very hard to make itself appear *all science*, and that meant subverting its spiritual element.

It is only recently that some educators have felt the absence of a spiritual element and have sought to reinstate it, first by inserting spirituality into nursing theory (as Chapter 6 illustrated) and then in curriculum content.

TEACHING SPIRITUALITY RATHER THAN RELIGION

Other than a very few schools owned by religious organizations, in recent years there has seldom been much religious content in nursing education and less that could be called spiritual. Inclusion of so-called spiritual elements often turned out to be sociological aspects of religion, usually dealing with religious cultural constraints such as dietary limitations, Hassidic formalities between men and women, what to do about Mormon underwear, and other such restrictions in religious codes. Hence, spirituality was often overlooked, and religion was reduced to the management of specific ritual dictates.

Notice the safety of this position. Surely, it is humanistic and merely good psychology to be respectful of a patient's religious beliefs and practices. One can do this without ever saying anything about the nurse's sense of the spiritual. Aha, we are still the scientists.

If we are going to teach spirituality instead of religion, we need to remind ourselves of the difference between these two areas (as seen in Chapter 1). Michael Grosso (2009) gives us a good reminder:

> A distinction is sometimes made between *religious* and *spiritual*. People say, "I'm not very religious, but I consider myself a spiritual person." Such a person is not likely to be attached to any mainline system of organized religion. The emphasis would be on unstructured, undogmatized openness to inward experience; and less, if at all, on the recitation of creeds, ritual behaviors, or anything that smacks of the mechanical and the pseudo-spiritual. (p. 9)

Grosso emphasizes the inward experience here, but most experts address both the inward and the outward elements of spirituality.

We often find issues of spirituality and religion mixed. The advice given to student nurses when an issue of spirituality arises is often to call the chaplain. In other words, nurses are told that both spirituality and religion are the turf of another profession.

Yet the question remains: If spirituality is different from religion, is there a separate domain of spirituality with its own experts? Who are the appropriate teachers of spirituality? Should nurses be part of this group?

Most schools will find that religious stewards of any group are likely to blur spirituality with religion. Often a teacher from the discipline of philosophy will be more evenhanded in managing a course in spirituality.

When nurse faculty wish to teach such a course, we often find their knowledge of the subject matter to be too limited. Look, for example, at Peter Van Ness's (1992) description of spirituality:

> What is spiritual is a specific aspect of human existence, one that has been hypothesized here to have an outer and inner complexion. Facing outward human existence has been deemed spiritual insofar as it intentionally engages reality as a maximally inclusive whole. Facing inward, life has been accorded a spiritual dimension to the extent that it has been experienced as a project of one's most vital and enduring self. And integration of these inner and outer characterizations is achieved by equating the spiritual dimension of life with the existential task of discovering one's truest self in the context of reality apprehended as a cosmic reality. (pp. 273–274)

One must ask, how many nurses can effectively teach a subject matter of this complexity that is not from their primary discipline? Moreover, how many nurses can teach such a complex subject matter without slipping in a religious ideology? Few will truly be prepared for this task.

SPIRITUALITY AS A NECESSARY ASPECT
IN NURSING EDUCATION

Despite the difficulties it presents, many would argue that we have sacrificed too much in eliminating spirituality from our nursing focus. First, nurses do face patients' spiritual crises and conflicts in clinical practice. Often there are no religious or spiritual experts available. Is it fair *not* to prepare students to deal with these spiritual issues? We would certainly not take on any other aspect of nursing care as casually as we take on spirituality nor with so little preparation.

HOW DO WE TEACH SPIRITUALITY?

When a nursing faculty seriously intends to teach spirituality, how can that be done? First, we must realize that teaching a subject whose outcome is a value appreciation is different from teaching a subject whose outcome is cognitive knowledge. Values are caught as much as taught.

Ironically, this is another reason that aspects of spirituality were removed from nursing curricula when we began our love affair with terminal objectives. Faculty didn't know how to construct values goals, and accrediting agencies didn't know how to handle them either. The easiest way apparently was to simply drop them from the curriculum.

Faculty had to differentiate between cognitive content and inculcating in students certain ways of thinking about spirituality and of dealing with patients who have spiritual problems. It was many years before most faculty felt comfortable inserting such subjects back into curriculum documents and teaching. Teaching content about spirituality is a challenge when our student nurses differ in both their conceptions of spirituality and their level of spiritual development.

WHAT IS INCULCATION?

Inculcation is a method of teaching that goes beyond providing information. It involves persistent teaching to implant certain values and behaviors in the learner. It is a method of influence designed to cause the learner to accept certain ideas, feelings, or values. Often the subject one wishes to cultivate in the learner involves social and moral values. A good role model may be more effective than numerous lectures. Yet the process of inculcation necessarily involves teaching content too.

One way around the complexity of inculcating values (in our case, the value of spirituality) is to use the teaching method of case studies. This is in contrast to the usual lectures that give principles first, followed by examples and applications. Case studies can embed spiritual problems in ambiguous situations that allow the student to extract the principles.

There are two obvious ways to apply this process. The first occurs in the student's clinical practice. The instructor puts the real spiritual crises that occur there into the form of clinical conferences. This way, many students learn from one student's problem encounter. Because spiritual issues occur in context, this is the logical way to use them as teaching moments.

Another approach is teaching spirituality through simulated case studies. These, of course, are as close as one can get to real clinical events. Indeed, collected case studies are often based on real events that happened to others. The situational approach of case studies starts all students on the same level, with the same data. A case then lends itself to exploring different options for action, which is extremely important for a subject matter where there is no single right answer.

Spirituality need not begin with its principles. Indeed, principles may vary with different conceptualizations of spirituality. Look at the irreconcilable differences between abortion/no abortion groups, between those using T-cells for research and application versus those refusing to use T-cells. Where there exists no agreed-upon beginning principles, it is better to let conclusions (even if they differ) arise from indeterminate situations. Then one can intellectually determine from where the conclusions were derived. This approach allows the students to grow in their perceptions of spiritual subtleties as they wrestle with the remarkable facts of real-life situations.

The case study approach also had the advantage of engaging students who are at different levels of spirituality. The more spiritually mature can help guide the less mature. Moreover, this helps retain the interest of both groups in the subject matter.

I have seen both of these approaches (real clinical cases and simulated case studies) work remarkably well with mixed groups of student nurses and medical students. Indeed, spirituality is a level playing field for this kind of coming together. No health care profession has an edge on others concerning spiritual quandaries.

ETHICS

One way that spirituality is sometimes slipped into a curriculum or in-service education is in the guise of ethics. Spirituality and ethics both have to do with what is right and wrong, but they connote different images and different ways of handling oneself in the world. Ethics has more to do with how people regulate their relationships with each other, whereas spirituality has more to do with one's relationship to God or to a perceived higher good.

Rules for ethical conduct evolve from the generally accepted mores of a culture. Ethics concerns situations where the nurse might do the wrong thing, with *wrong* defined as something that may have legal consequences. Medical ethics asks how to manage health-related problems when people disagree over the right action. In contrast, spirituality relates to the joyous experience of soul growth and connection with a higher good.

Circumstances, among others, that lead to issues of medical ethics involve:

1. New technologies that influence the meaning of human life (e.g., new ways of creating, sustaining, or ending human life or therapies arising from stem cell research)
2. Issues of resource scarcity (e.g., present discussions of vast and usu-ally futile resources devoted to the events surrounding incipient death of geriatric patients)
3. Increasing sensitivity to human rights (e.g., can parents legally refuse the use of now available therapy for children with cancer)

Ethics clearly puts us in the world of making judgments, decisions that often involve issues of law. Ethical quandaries arise in situations that demand the selection of a single answer, when concrete choices must be made.

Perhaps the best way to understand ethics is to see how it is approached as an intellectual subject—usually in the field of philosophy. Figure 7.1 illus-trates one such approach.

This illustration parses ethics according to an operational (either/or) design as discussed in Chapter 5. As the schema in Figure 7.1 indicates, a decision made at any level dictates the choices available at the next level below. The diagram also shows why good people can disagree on ethical issues.

The first differentiation in this illustration is between philosophies of *determinism* and human *freedom*. In determinism, things happen in terms of antecedents. If one knew all the events and experiences that had happened in his or her past, one could predict the present course of action of a person. In this belief system, there is no such thing as free will. One's choices are determined by what happened earlier. Hence, in this philosophy, any sense of choice is an illusion. Yet if all choices are the inevitable results of earlier events, there can't actually be ethical or moral accountability. Ethics is an illusory study.

To allow for ethics, there must first be some freedom of choice, the ability to choose right over wrong. Hence, the rest of our branching philosophy falls

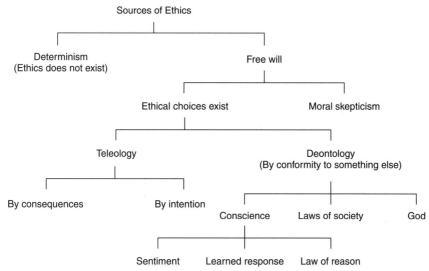

FIGURE 7.1 Why Good People Disagree on Ethical Issues

within the concept of human freedom. Even where freedom is espoused, there are alternate positions. In *moral skepticism*, people choose, but they are not guided by ethical positions. Moral choice is illusory; ethics is an empty word. People choose for other reasons, primarily self-interest. Of course, choices may be dressed up as ethical, but beneath the surface, self-interest reveals itself.

The position of *ethical choice* grants that a human being can make a choice based on ethical considerations. Yet in this case, there is another basic discrimination: between *teleological* and *deontological* positions. Teleology is driven by the perceived goal or outcome. Teleological systems assert that people choose based on what will happen, given their decisions.

Within teleological positions, another determination point occurs. Here one asks, what makes a choice ethical? Its eventual *outcome* or its *intention*? The first position resting in the *outcome*, of course, assumes that one has the capacity to predict the results of given actions—or at least assumes that one can predict the most likely outcomes. In outcome-driven teleology, the result is the total arbiter of whether a choice was ethical. So if a choice produces an unexpected, negative outcome, then the choice is labeled unethical.

The second position, resting on *intentions*, recognizes the fact that predicted intentions don't always lead to the anticipated outcome. How often we hear, "He meant well." Moreover, here the intention is where the right or wrong judgment rests. Results don't matter; the ethics rest in intention. Hence, teleological ethical systems may be judged by either intentions or actual outcomes.

Go back up the grid to the *deontological* choice, and we find that deontology does not make ethical judgments based on any aspect of outcomes (neither intention nor consequences). Instead, a different set of variables appears depending on that to which the choice conforms. Three of the most common options are *conscience*, *laws of society*, and *God* (or his revealed word).

When one begins with conscience, the difficulties are quickly evident because not all consciences provide the same answer. (Recall abortion vs. anti-abortion advocates.) Only the criterion of conscience (*let your conscience be your guide*) is elaborated in the diagram, but one can easily imagine the other options providing equal complexity. Under the criterion of conscience, we find three more branching options: *sentiment, learned response*, and the *law of reason* (and these are only the most common three).

With *sentiment*, the inner voice might be the referent, that is, whatever *feels* right. In the case of nursing, this criterion might refer us clear back to Florence Nightingale, who claimed to actually hear an *inner voice*.

A *learned response* might be represented by what one has been taught in one's society (e.g., what one's superego sees as good in a Freudian system). Culturally indoctrinated suicide bombers also might fall in this category. Obviously, a learned response can be traced back to societal indoctrination.

Finally, the *law of reason* might involve dictates such as Kant's *categorical imperative*. Kant claimed that one must act in such a way that the rest of humankind could perform the very same act. This, would, for example, rule out euthanasia because I could not trust the rest of humankind to make rational decisions in every other case subjected to a decision concerning euthanasia.

Hence, as this diagram illustrates, ethics deals with the scientific study of moral choices. Although recognizing different ethical stances is very important, it is an intellectual approach to morality. Certainly, it may invoke one's sense of the spiritual, but one can easily study ethics from a removed perspective, without involving any sense of spirituality.

SUMMARY

No amount of teaching about ethics is enough to make one spiritual. Ethics is an intellectual approach to right and wrong. However, one's spirituality, which might (or might not) be strengthened by such understanding, is based on one's unique sense of ultimate meaning. Nurses can be given content related to spirituality, but they may not *catch* the context that gives spirituality meaning. Role modeling becomes more important than education in many cases: inspiration over education.

The chronological age of the practicing nurse becomes equally important as we saw in Chapter 2. As Fowler realized, on the whole, people advance in stages of faith as they mature in other aspects of growth and development. This, of course, does not apply in every case. However, on the whole, a group of older nurses will be more spiritually mature than a group of younger nurses. As our student population ages (which is happening at present), we may have fewer spiritually immature nurses.

If spirituality is a developmental stage, nursing has not in our lifetime required a certain level of spiritual development as a criterion for entrance into its programs of education. And, unfortunately, persons in various stages of development tend to think that their own particular stage is the important one, not seeing beyond the inculcated beliefs at their present level of spiritual growth.

Nurses today come from many different cultures, complete with many different value systems. Hence, nurses need, more than ever, to separate issues of spirituality and religion. The study of spirituality, because it is less confined and regimented than religion, is a more appropriate subject matter for our multicultural student body.

These are a few of the challenges that arise when spirituality is made part of a curriculum. Yet can we fail to include in a curriculum an element that is certain to rear its head when a student graduates?

REFERENCES

Grosso, M. (2009, Summer). What is spirituality? In *PsychoSpiritual Dialogue* (pp. 9–11). New York: Association for Spirituality and Psychotherapy.

Van Ness, P. H. (1992). *Spirituality, diversion, and decadence: The contemporary predicament.* Albany, NY: State University of New York Press.

CHAPTER 8

Spirituality, Healing, and Nursing: Should Nursing Claim Healing as Part of Its Mission?

Healing presents a peculiar quandary for nursing but not a new one. Nursing has frequently taken on methods of care that are shared with other professions or that ultimately are taken over as new separate professions that then lay claim to these processes—sometimes exclusive claim. Respiratory therapy and massage therapy represent only two of the methods that have gone this direction over the years. Indeed, one of the major challenges in nursing is that it often becomes the home of techniques that are then spun into separate professions or occupations.

Nursing cannot claim to be the first profession to take on healing. Indeed, healing has a long historical connection to religion through the process of the *laying on of hands*. Yet it has gained nursing acceptance in the domain of holistic nursing. Indeed, nursing has claimed its own process of healing under the rubric of *Therapeutic Touch*.

How do we handle a method that is not and never will be strictly a nursing method? Although healing is associated with our interest in spirituality, the issue of shared methods remains a challenge for nursing. The information below will serve to bring the reader up to date on the specifics of healing methods, related physiology, and its present status.

Nursing has always had an interest in healing. By this, I mean healing as a technique of its own not as the eventual outcome of multiple traditional cure treatments. All nursing and all medicine aim at healing in general, but here we'll discuss the more direct forms of healing that are thought to pass directly from one person (the healer) to another (the patient/client).

In nursing, the interest in healing as a technique has been associated primarily with holistic nursing practice, and the usually favored technique of healing is *Therapeutic Touch*. Nursing has applied this label to techniques that are essentially like healing practices in other fields, namely, processes that deal with energy work—transmitting energy, moving energy, or even removing excess energy from the client. Usually, the energy movement is through the healer's hands.

Although energy transfer in this manner is the usual modality, there also are assertions that the process may occur spontaneously in normal interpersonal relationships. For example, the simplest form of healing may be found in Barbara Dossey's (Dossey, Keegan, Guzzetta, & Kolkmeier, 1995) view of *being* as applied to nursing. She differentiates between two kinds of nursing acts: being and doing. Being has to do with the healing effects of the nurse just being there, beyond what she does in her normal care routines. This form of being is also noted by Barbara Brennan (1987). She says that we all manipulate each other's energy fields in the course of our daily lives, regardless of whether we realize it.

We recognize this simple form of healing when it happens, and we recognize its absence as well. For example, a patient who unexpectedly survived recounted an event that happened to him in Intensive Care after open-heart surgery. The patient, who also suffered from leukemia, was apparently not fighting off a MRSA infection. He was intubated, on a ventilator, on dialysis, and also suffering from what turned out to be a temporary hearing loss. His body was virtually tied down by various intravenous and monitoring lines. His wife had refused to sign the *Do Not Resuscitate* forms given to her. She and his original cardiologist held out against this logical step proposed by his surgeons.

In any case, the patient, now recuperated, recalls during this time when he was too weak and incapacitated to communicate, a male nurse taking care of his physical body, then turning on the television set to a ballgame, which gave the patient a moment of welcome pleasure. But then, the nurse pulled up a chair at the end of the bed, turned his back to the patient, and placed himself where he could watch the game, his own body positioned where it blocked the patient's view of the screen. Here is a nurse who will always be remembered for his total lack of sensitivity to the notion of *being there* for the patient.

For the rest of this chapter, however, we address the more intensive view of healing, one in which the nurse creates a direct connection that intentionally sends healing energy from the nurse to the patient. Most commonly, this form of healing is described in terms of an energic (energy) exchange. In many cases, the person applying these techniques claims to receive direction from some internal guidance or from some external source, often described as the patient's or the nurse's guides, teachers, and/or angels. In other cases, the nurse claims to be drawing energy up through his/her body from a universal energy source.

Most nurses and other healers have incorporated, along with their healing techniques, some sense of the spiritual. As one such healer, Louisiana Zinn, a Reiki Master, (2002) reports:

> When one is out of harmony or balance with the divine source of energy (the light), disharmony or dis-ease is created. When one's body is attuned to Reiki, there is an immediate ability to channel unlimited living light energy and to facilitate healing on a very deep level. (p. 70)

It is impossible to read even this one paragraph without seeing how embedded the healer's practice is in a spiritual philosophy of life. In this case, a belief that is set apart from attachment to any particular religion. The Reiki tradition, indeed, claims itself to be separate from religion. Yet it rests in a clear spiritual vision of the nature of reality.

In nursing, the healing adaptation (typically Therapeutic Touch) has been heavily weighed in terms of touch on the body or movement of the healer's hands directly above the body. This, of course, is a practice that is shared with the much older religious practice referred to as *laying on of hands*. Today there are many different forms of energy work in this tradition.

Some practitioners of healing claim to be able to contact a person's discarnate (or spiritual) guides and teachers, sometimes visible to the healer in the person's immediate environment. Many healers agree upon the existence of these personal guides and teachers. Barbara Brennan (1987), a nonnurse who also uses energy work delivered through the hands above or on the body, says:

> Each person has several guides who stay with him and guide him throughout many lifetimes. In addition, one has teacher-guides who stay during times of specific learning and are chosen because of that specific learning. (p. 171)

Although healers who see such guides agree on this source of healing assistance, there is less evidence to confirm agreement as to the identity of any subject's specific guides. Different healers seeing the same client may describe quite different guides and teachers.

It is difficult to find credible studies validating commonalities seen by different healers describing the same persons under controlled conditions. In a different study of psychic abilities, Gary Schwartz with William Simon (2002) produced some rather positive research where different psychics read the same subjects concerning their deceased friends and relatives. This study may come closest to providing some data on comparing different readings of psychic phenomena for the same subject.

Inconsistencies among interpretations do not necessarily invalidate the gifts of healers but may indicate that the perceptions of healers are more complicated than they appear. There is considerable agreement that what is seen and/or interpreted is filtered through the healer's own personal character and beliefs.

CLAIMED CONNECTIONS

Nor do all healers see or sense spiritual helpers. In some energy systems, including Reiki and Therapeutic Touch, that is not required. Yet many healers receive auditory, sensate, or visual information. Some healers allow discarnate entities (deceased persons or spiritual teachers) to borrow their bodies to speak through their vocal cords or at least to be heard internally by the healer. Indeed, so popular is *channeling*, as it is called, that it has almost become a parlor game.

A healer such as Edgar Cayce (e.g., Lytle Robinson, 1972; Jeffrey Furst, 1982) represents one extreme in channeling. Cayce, while in an unconscious trance state, was taken over by a noncorporeal entity who gave health therapy prescriptions for thousands. When Cayce returned from an altered state, he had no memory of these messages. Cayce, a man without any medical training, was also faced with his own spiritual crisis. Initially, his early fundamentalist religion gave him grave doubts about his trance-generated materials.

Many modern healers work in a lighter trance that allows them to remain conscious, communicating with a discarnate entity and reporting what was conveyed. L. Austin (personal communication, 2010), a nurse healer, illustrates this application. In personal correspondence, Lynne revealed a spontaneous event with a shamanic orientation and an added element of channeling:

> While a client was on my table receiving body work, I suddenly began to hear thoughts in my head which weren't mine. He (the client) was in a place this day, of feeling stressed and overwhelmed. The words that were coming to me were addressing his life. I began to speak the words I was hearing, wondering if the words would make sense. The words made perfect sense to him. The words moved him and gave him great peace. At the very end of the advice, he was given a name to call himself. The name was Clear Eagle.
>
> He was in awe of the advice, but more so of the name given to him. He related that not long before this session, a good friend had sent him a gift out of the blue. She had said, "I don't know why I am sending this to you, but when I saw it, I thought of you. So I bought it." It was a clear glass eagle.

Although Lynne was channeling the words of another entity, she was not *possessed* by it; that is, she never lost consciousness of herself and she never gave up control of her body. It was the nature of the name, Clear Eagle, that ties this experience to Lynne's shamanic tradition. Indeed, the eagle is a powerful totem and often involved in shamanic shape shifting.

Lynne Austin (2002) also surprisingly found herself being guided to use sound as a healing tool, even treating cancer with specific directed sounds. She describes how she became a sound therapist:

> . . . I knew instinctively that each organ of our body vibrates to a particular resonance, and if we could only find that vibration, we could begin curing disease and bringing harmony to the body. (p. 27)

> . . . I began to intuit more sounds and tones when my clients were on the table . . .
>   The next two years took me on a journey of discovery of my abilities, the courage to use those abilities and the use of sound with all my clients. . . . (p. 28)

According to many, the lighter trance state is ultimately easier on the healer. Most psychics, in describing the phenomenon of reaching discarnate beings of any sort, speak of a difference in the level of vibration between people or entities embodied on earth and discarnate ones. Often the psychic speaks of raising his vibrations to be able to effect the contact. Others speak of the discarnate being lowering his vibrations at the same time. Because different healers may tune into different vibrational levels, it is not surprising that they may have diverse perceptions.

Many healers find themselves contacting beings from other dimensions of reality at some stage in their healing practice. Yet other branches of energy movement claim that healing can occur entirely by intention and that such extra perception is not essential. These schools believe that the energy delivered by the healer is all that is required.

RELIGIOUS AND SPIRITUAL BELIEFS OF HEALERS

Most healers develop a metaphysical interpretation of reality, which by its nature has a spiritual essence. In 2002, I wrote a book examining nine healers on various aspects of their work and beliefs. Of the group, four were nurses. These nine healers, who all happened to be women, worked with techniques of herbology, sound therapy, astrology, neurofeedback, thought field therapy, Reiki, rolfing, craniosacral therapy, acupuncture, essential oil therapy, and shamanic practice, among others.

One of the categories addressed in my questions to them concerned their religion and spiritual beliefs. Although this sample was small, their answers seemed in context with the many other healers I have met. Nevertheless, the reader should keep in mind that my findings represent only a small sample.

Some of the healers I interviewed belonged to a traditional religion, but their beliefs were usually broader than the usual religious context. Others held no specific religion but claimed to hold spiritual beliefs. Even those who practiced a given religion did not hold closely to dogma.

Yet three of the healers were ordained ministers in what happened to be three different denominations (Protestant or Interfaith). Most healers held a blending of elements from various faiths, and most had a great tolerance for patients' different beliefs. Whatever their *official* religions, most believed that they tapped into a Universal Energy Source for healing.

Most of these healers used what I called a religious supermarket approach in their beliefs. For example, in her work, one frequently called on Jesus, Sai Baba, and Quan Yin. Another who was raised Catholic also worked with principles of Zen Buddhism and Taoism. Another combined shamanism and calling on Jesus.

In essence, the healers tended to be very interested in different religions and spiritual paths while picking and choosing elements that appealed to them or felt applicable to their work. The supermarket mentality applied to the ministers as well as the others. Indeed, all the healers tended to be very comfortable with diverse perceptions, feeling that all these different paths led ultimately back to the one same Source. This flexibility made it possible for them to work comfortably with clients from many different belief systems.

ENERGIC CONCEPTS

Energic healers channel a perceived universal energy (prana) or use their personal energy to heal. Several terms are used for this art: energy work, energetic healing, energic healing, or bioenergetics. Energy workers manipulate the client's energy field by adding, subtracting, or balancing energy. The energic system is seen as a subtle and separate component of the total body/mind system.

Some researchers and health field experts question the existence of this energy system. Whatever the reality, energic healers believe that they manipulate their own energy, a client's energy, and/or a purported universal energy for the purpose of healing. Depending on their vision, their notion of reality and their education, energic healers manipulate various layers of the person's energy being (i.e., aural layers) as well as the physical body.

For the rest of this discussion we'll assume the therapy involves movement of the energic factor by transmission through the healer's hands. Obviously, however, some use sound, energy of the mind (healing at a distance), and other means of moving energy. Before manipulating a client's energy field, the healer typically uses a ritual of centering himself—apart from external influences, drawing on sources of power, and using intentionality to direct the energy to the client. These acts, especially the centering, probably induce a light state of altered consciousness in the healer.

Brennan tries to explain energic healing on a basis that is compatible with the physical sciences. She claims that what she calls *High Sense Perception* directs the healer's actions. As she describes it, High Sense Perception involves a psychic perception (be it sight, somatic sense, or some other perception).

Reiki practitioners, using a somewhat different method of energy movement, claim that the key lies in the practitioner's upper chakras (energy vortices) being open. Whatever the criterion, it is probable that the effective practitioner enters a psychic, spiritual, or alternate state of consciousness in order to move energy.

Another healer, Victoria Slater (Part I, 1955a) describes the healer's work as intervening in the client's chaotic energy system:

> The task of the practitioner is to continue infusing energy until a new, non-chaotic pattern can be detected, which often is sensed as a calm, organized, and gliding flow of energy. Once chaos has evolved into a new form, the treatment is over. (p. 221)

Although Brennan treats this energy as a physical fact of life, Slater hedges by calling it a metaphor rather than asserting that her model is an actual physiological prototype. Energy healers disagree on just how energy is to be moved, what degree of perception is necessary on the part of the practitioner before he can be effective, and on just what happens during the purported movement of energy. Nevertheless, most energy healers work from a description of the human energy field that is in concert with the patterns described here.

Energy workers usually grant that some untrained people have an instinctive ability to move energy, but most would not grant that moving of one's hands over a patient's body without the appropriate mind set, or without knowledgeable control of energies, could be effective except serendipitously. The issue is twofold: (1) whether the attempt to manipulate energy can be effective apart from extensive training with verification of what the practitioner is doing and (2) whether the healer must have attained certain levels of personal development and/or a requisite state of consciousness in which to exercise the skill.

However, most energy workers describe four major steps: (1) centering oneself, so that one is detached from outside interference, thoughts, or negativities; (2) grounding oneself in an energy source outside of oneself in such a way that one can tap that universal energy; (3) focusing that energy through oneself into the client so as not to draw on one's own bodily energy; and

(4) exercising intentionality, that is, employing the will and affect so as to intend a good effect.

In a slightly different formulation, Barbara Dossey, Lynn Keegan, Cathie Guzzetta, and Leslie Kolkmeier (1995) describe the phases of *Therapeutic Touch* as centering oneself, assessing the client with sensitive hands, mobilizing stagnant areas in the client's energy field, and providing energy to repattern the client's energy.

Energy movement techniques are not so much different as is the interpretation of what is happening. In a religious context, *laying on of hands* is seen as conveying God's power and will through the healer. Other practices of energic movement are often conceptualized as manipulating a universal power. Some see movement of these energies as purely physiological; others claim to be working on a subtle level of energy that is not physiological in origin (discussed later in this chapter).

There are many different schools of energic healing, each with its own techniques and its own ideology. Most see the healer's hands as the primary transmittal tools. Some schools prefer that touch occur between practitioner and client; others believe that energic healing can take place without touch and that distance between the healer and the client is irrelevant. Some think energy is always sent to the client; others think the objective is energy balance, that is, energy infusion, rearrangement, or energy release. Some schools think the practitioner must perceive the energy flow; some don't.

As indicated earlier, energy practitioners vary in the degree to which vision enters their work. Some see and feel nothing; most feel the energy in their hands or in the client's body. Yet others claim that they see the client's aural layers and deficits created by disease processes. In addition, as mentioned earlier, some will see guides and spirits who indicate what the healer should do for the client.

Clients also vary in what they perceive during the treatment. A few claim to have seen the noncorporeal guides; many simply feel energy changes in their bodies. Others have few perceptions during the treatment but feel results thereafter.

THE SUBTLE HUMAN ENERGY SYSTEM

The subtle human energy system (probably the system drawn upon by energy healers) is *not* the nervous system of the physical body. Indeed, this energy system has yet to be acknowledged in Western medicine. What is the nature of this energy system? John Pierrakos (1987) ponders this very question:

> I found myself more and more concerned with the nature and innate functioning of the life force itself. I wondered: What is this energy? Is it both

substance and attribute . . .? Is it universal spirit, individualized somehow in matter . . .? Is it essentially material . . .? Is it essentially spiritual . . .? (p. 13)

The questions Pierrakos raises have yet to be answered. However this energy system is defined, it is not located in the physical body and hence not traceable in medical studies limited to the anatomy and physiology of the visible body. If it is in the physical body, it has not yet been found and measured.

In general, healers who work with the *human energy field* describe it as a body or bodies surrounding and penetrating the physical body. Some healers see this body as a surrounding aura, some sense it, for example, with their hands. Some see or feel one layer, some are able to discriminate many layers. Nik Douglas and Penny Slinger (2000) call this system the subtle body and describe it this way:

> Esoteric teachings contend that men and women have an "auric" or Subtle Body as well as a physical body. Normally the various life energies in the body generate a kind of subtle "field" or aura, which can be seen by sensitives. (p. 30)

However, the subtle human energy system is described; two elements of the system receive particular attention: the chakras and Kundalini energy. In addition, the status of the chakras is often seen by those able to do so, in visible auric layers surrounding the body.

THE CHAKRA ENERGY VORTICES

The chakras are vortices or centers that regulate energy intake and release in the body. Different authors claim that the body has different numbers of major chakras, usually ranging from seven to ten. Chakras can be found in various states of efficiency, from being closed to fully open. Opening these channels wider (or opening closed ones) changes the energy quotient of the body. Smaller chakras exist throughout the body. Reiki masters claim that they open various higher chakras of initiates, allowing the initiate to better access universal energy. If there is validity to these claims concerning chakras, then the healer may have become *child-like* in the sense of having open chakras that afford a greater intake of psychic phenomena at the potential cost of greatly increased vulnerability to psychic infringements.

Many claim that children's chakras are less protected and that this may account for their enhanced capacities for various psychic perceptions. If this is true, we may need to rethink the origin of many of their *imaginary* friends.

People differ on how many layers the associated aura around the body contains. Brennan associates the number of layers observed with the development of the healer (what he/she is able to perceive) rather than with variations among how many layers actually comprise a human being. With experience, healers learn to interpret what they see in these energic layers. The usual sight refers to colors, often with so-called muddy patches over areas of physical problems.

KUNDALINI ENERGY

Kundalini energy is the most discussed current in the subtle human energy system, primarily because it is the flow most likely to be perceived. Kundalini energy, called the serpent power, is supposed to lie curled around the base of the spine, rising through the body chakras once activated. Typically, Kundalini is described as ascending the spine, although there are accounts of it moving down the spine as well.

Arousing the Kundalini power is a goal of some Hindu and Buddhist Tantric practices, particularly those that use sexual performance as a spiritual practice. Here male practitioners are sometimes taught to substitute a Kundalini experience in place of ejaculation. The Kundalini energy can be awakened by various spiritual or prescribed yogic states. It can also be an unanticipated side effect of spiritual development.

Lilian Silburn (1988) describes Kundalini as universal energy, as:

> . . . the source of all rhythms in life; what it generates is nothing but rhythm, and no level escapes it. . . . So the Kundalini energy is nothing but vibration—the vibrant undulation of emanation, the more and more subtle vibration of resorption—a high frequency vibration. (pp. 5–6)

Appropriate energy flow brings pleasurable sensations; however, inappropriate flow can be disabling and painful. Kundalini may be responsible for either pleasure or considerable pain. Indeed, uncontrolled Kundalini energy may incapacitate the person experiencing it. Gopi Krishna (1993) gives a personal account of problems arising with the awakening of the Kundalini energy (repeated here in part):

> The moment my head touched the pillow a large tongue of flame sped across the spine into the interior of my head. It appeared as if the stream of living light continuously rushing through the spinal cord into the cranium gathered greater speed and volume during the hours of darkness. (p. 145)

The awakening of the Kundalini current can be so physically painful as to cause many bodily and emotional problems, sometimes causing the person to virtually lose years of his life. Stanislav and Chistina Grof (1990) list it as one of the common spiritual emergencies. Clearly Kundalini energy is a two-edged sword of potential delight or potential torture.

Arguments concerning the source of Kundalini follow the same paths as arguments concerning the nature of the rest of the subtle energy system. In the edited work of Carl Jung, Sonu Shamdasani (1996) claims that Jung views Kundalini primarily as a psychological phenomenon. In this translation, Jung describes Kundalini as: ". . . a purely theoretic abstraction. The Western mind can do nothing with it. To the Indian way of thinking such hypostatized abstractions are much more concrete and substantial" (p. 69).

Different methods are said to result in awakening Kundalini, including meditation, often with given mantras; yoga, with particular body positions; breathing techniques; and other techniques associated with awakening psychic, mystic, or spiritual abilities.

SUMMARY

If we return to our original question, we must ask if nursing gains by keeping healing in its armamentarium of methods. It clearly is a method that must be shared with other fields, particularly since it did not originate in nursing and has never been solely attributed to nursing. Yet it is a method in keeping with many of the principles of holistic nursing.

There are several things to consider with healing. First, the practice is presently questioned by many health professionals. Yet there is considerable agreement among healers on the existence of an energy system that is, as yet, unidentified in modern physiological research. The subtle human energy system is said to use chakras as energy vortices. Kundalini energy is one of the chief energy channels of the system. Energy healers claim to be manipulating aspects of this subtle human energy system for clients' healing.

Yet there is no doubt that others in the field of health care, particularly physicians, will take exception to this method. Clearly, this is not the first challenge to medicine's hold on the ideology of health care. One remembers physician's initial resistance to acupuncture, for example, as another historical challenge. There are both advantages and disadvantages for nursing in using techniques that challenge medical thinking. One of our greatest gains (many nurse practitioner roles) has been in the domain that is in concert with medicine's ideology. Is there adequate space for the challenge that healing presents to this status quo?

Another challenge to the use of healing by nurses comes from religious sources, especially when some nurses see it primarily as a physiological/energic method apart from its spiritual origins. Nevertheless, most healers, nurses among them, cast their healing practice in both an energic context and a spiritual context. For many healers, the spiritual aspect is intrinsic to their work. Yet their religious and/or spiritual beliefs typically are flexible and tolerant. Perhaps part of their flexibility concerning beliefs along with the strong spiritual values they hold arise from the fact that these spiritual elements are so intertwined in the rest of the healers' lives.

Yet this is not always true of nurses who practice healing. Some view it as separate from any spiritual connection—simply as an energic process. Nurses who eschew the spiritual connection will be challenged by religious sources who look upon healing as a spiritual endeavor.

Healing is deeply entrenched in holistic nursing, and it is highly probable that it will remain there. Yet we need to be aware of the vulnerabilities that arise in making this a nursing method.

REFERENCES

Austin, L. (2010). Personal communication.

Austin, L. (2002). Interview: Lynne Austin, sound therapist. In B. Barnum, *The new healers: Minds and hands in complementary medicine* (pp. 24–36). Long Beach, NJ: Vista Publishing.

Barnum, B. (2002). *The new healers: Minds and hands in complementary medicine.* Long Beach, NJ: Vista Publishing.

Brennan, B. A. (1987). *Hands of light: A guide to healing through the human energy field.* New York: Bantam Books.

Douglas, N. & Slinger, P. (2000). *Sexual secrets: The alchemy of ecstasy* (20th anniversary ed.). Rochester, VT: Destiny Books.

Krishna, G. (1993). *Living with Kundalini.* Boston: Shambhala.

Pierrakos, J. C. (1987). *Core energetics: Developing the capacity to love and heal.* Mendocino, CA: Life Rhythm Publication.

Shamdasani, S. (Ed.). (1996). *The psychology of Kundalini yoga: Notes of the seminar given in 1932 by C. G. Jung.* Princeton, NJ: Princeton University Press.

Silburn, L. (1988). *Kundalini: Energy of the depths.* Albany, NY: State University of New York Press.

Slater, V. E. (1995a). Toward an understanding of energetic healing, Part 1. *Journal of Holistic Nursing,* 13(3): 209–224.

Zinn, L. (2002). Interview: Louisiana Zinn, traditional Reiki master. In B. Barnum, *The new healers: Minds and hands in complementary medicine* (pp. 646–671). Long Beach, NJ: Vista Publishing.

BIBLIOGRAPHY

Austin, L. (2000). *Earth spirituality: Spiritual storytelling* (CD). Waukesha, WI: Singing Bear Productions.

Dossey, B. M., Keegan, L., Guzzetta, C. E., & Kolkmeier, L. G. (1995). *Holistic nursing: A handbook for practice* (2nd ed.). Gaithersburg, MD: Aspen Publishers.

Furst, J. (Ed.). (1982). *Edgar Cayce's story of attitudes and emotions*. New York: Berkley Books.

Grof, S., & Grof, C. (1990). *The stormy search for the self*. Los Angeles: Jeremy P. Tarcher, Inc.

Robinson, L. (1972). *Edgar Cayce's story of the origin and destiny of man*. New York: Berkley Books.

Schwartz, G. E., & Simon, W. L. (2002). *The afterlife experiments: Breakthrough scientific evidence of life after death*. New York: Pocket Books.

Slater, V. E. (1995b). Toward an understanding of energetic healing, Part 2. *Journal of Holistic Nursing*, 13(3): 225–238.

CHAPTER 9

Should Spiritual Care
Be a Function of Nursing
Practice?

Is spiritual care a legitimate nursing function? Is it logical to expect nurses to incorporate aspects of spirituality into patient care? Should nurses deal with patients' spiritual dilemmas? Alternatively, do they have any choice?

Even if we were to remove spiritual care from the nursing role, nurses will still find themselves in situations where they must deal with spiritual issues. Existential crises occur in the hot bed of caring for clients. Patients suddenly ask questions about spiritual matters or make pronouncements with good or bad spiritual implications.

Then practical questions arise, such as:

1. How can nurses who themselves are at relatively immature levels of spiritual development give spiritual care to more advanced patients?
2. How can the nurse figure out the spiritual needs of patients if spirituality is unique for each individual?
3. How can the nurse assist the patient if these two have entirely different images and orientations of spirituality or religion (a common event in our multicultural society)?

These are not easy questions to answer, especially when most nurses are ill prepared to deal with the spiritual values of other people. Seldom are nurses prepared in nursing education programs or in in-service education.

SPIRITUALITY: DEFINITIONS

Once again, let's remind ourselves of the differences between religion and spirituality. Let's use the conclusions of Alex Harris, Carl Thoresen, Michael McCullough, and David Larson (1999), who summarized their definitions after examining many authors. To paraphrase, they say that spirituality refers to a person's orientation toward, or experiences with, transcendent or existential phenomena. That is, spirituality refers to meaning, direction, purpose, and connectedness to the sacred. Spirituality is internal, affective, spontaneous, and private.

In contrast, they define religion as denominational, external, cognitive, and ritualistic behavior. Religion is primarily an external manifestation of spiritual experiences. They also note, as indicated earlier, that spirituality may be an attribute of religion or, at the opposite extreme, may even be antireligious.

When the patient persuades the nurse to share spiritual content, she/he might want to think about Michael Grosso's (2009) suggestion that there are two viewpoints on spirituality that are not in conflict. Regarding the first, he says:

> Spirituality often involves dramatic shifts in consciousness, moments of insight that result from unusual experiences. Sometimes drastic loss, trauma, or close encounters, mental or physical, with death may trigger such conversions. (p. 10)

Nurses see many dramatic responses like this in health care situations simply because they work in a domain of trauma, suffering, death, and permanent loss. Near-death encounters may represent the most dramatic spiritual events that a nurse observes. However, other stimuli may lead to dramatic spiritual shifts in consciousness as well. Such shifts may present many problems, often with family who have difficulty with what seems like a major personality change in the patient. Patients seldom go through such a dramatic spiritual shift without reaching out to others to help explain, or merely to hear, what has happened to them.

Yet as Grosso notes, not all spiritual experiences are so dramatic:

> But spiritual values may be explored in ordinary, everyday life, without drama or fanfare, and we may slowly and gradually cultivate such values. To begin with, it seems correct to honor with the word *spiritual,* the love of justice, of truth, and of beauty. (p. 10)

Nurses also see patients of this second sort: patients who are struggling to make sense of their altered lives. Often the nurse is the one who is sought as the patient tries to sort out even these gradual shifts in spiritual meaning.

COMMON SPIRITUAL PROBLEMS

Nurses are faced with many spiritual problems, most of them in a form that reflects the patient's spiritual dilemma. Perhaps the most common include:

1. Why me? What have I done to deserve this?
2. I'm overwhelmed; I can't cope.
3. Why did this happen? What is the message? What is this disease/injury saying to me? What is God trying to tell me?
4. I don't want to live with this disease and/or this suffering. There is nothing left but to die.
5. I'm afraid to die. I don't think there is anything after this life.
6. I'm afraid to die because I deserve to be punished by God.
7. I look forward to death; it will be so much better than this life. There is wonder on the other side of this journey. Why are you keeping me here?

However they cast their questions, patients are often thrown into spiritual dilemmas by the traumas of illness, injury, or incipient death. These existential circumstances may force them into spiritual inquiries.

DIFFERENT ORIENTATIONS

The issue of different spiritual orientations often creates a gulf between a patient and his nurse. This happens because, without broad knowledge and experience, the nurse is likely to assume that everyone thinks as he/she does. Worse, the nurse is likely to assume this without ever giving it a thought.

An example that comes to my mind is one I observed where such an assumption occurred internally—*within* a nurse rather than between nurse and patient. This nurse had come out of an order where she had been a nun for about 10 years. She thought she was ready for something less restrictive. Fowler might say she was stretching from Level 3 spiritual maturity toward Level 4.

In any case, she joined a Buddhist community where, every time she protested to the leader that he was failing to tell her what to do, he told her (once again) to go meditate on it. She never *got it* that the Buddhist orientation depended on gaining self-insight. She may have felt that she was ready for a less restrictive spiritual encounter, but without giving it any thought, she was still seeking the top-down directives of her prior religious training. She needed some authority figure to direct her. Finally, she left the Buddhist community, very bitter that no one would tell her what to do.

My point is that understanding a difference in spiritual context requires extensive analytic skills. This nurse was simply confused by the different orientation. If this nurse was unable to recognize her own assumptions, imagine how much difficulty she might have trying to recognize those of a patient. Failures here offer a great opportunity for misunderstanding between a nurse and a patient when they see issues of spirituality from different contexts.

PATIENT EXPECTATIONS

Although students usually can turn spiritual crises over to practicing nurses or faculty, nursing staff seldom have such a luxury. Patients present their spiritual crises to the nurses who regularly take care of them. Because of the nature of the environment where patients receive care, most spiritual issues occur as crises: crises of faith, crises of disillusion, crises of shock, and crises of understanding.

Spiritual crises often follow when patients (or significant others) are still in a state of disbelief concerning what has happened to them. Patients often feel that they have been betrayed by their bodies or by their spiritual expectations. As one woman said to me, "My body turned against me." Breast cancer turned this normally spiritual woman into two people: herself and her traitorous body. Nor was her path back to unity an easy journey.

Many patients are moved into spiritual crises because agreements they thought were held with higher powers turned out to be illusions. Then the patient's entire belief system may be vulnerable. What happens when patients lose their most significant interpretation of reality, their notion of God, and their perceived relationship with the forces of the universe?

Nurses face many challenges that span beyond the normal scope of their role. When there is no respiratory therapist available, the nurse becomes one. When a baby precipitates and there is no obstetrician available, she delivers it. When a physical therapist is not available, the nurse manages the follow-up daily exercises. When the patient experiences a spiritual crisis and no spiritual or religious leader is available, again the nurse is pressed into service.

Of all the examples given here, the spiritual care may be the situation for which the nurse is least prepared. At least the nurse knows the physiology of the human body and has probably seen the therapies required in the other cases. Seldom, however, has he or she observed the intimate one-on-one spiritual counseling offered by a minister, priest, or other spiritual professional. The issue is further confounded when the patient is spiritual but not religious.

There may be religious chaplains available, but they may not be right for the nonreligious person in spiritual crisis.

As in the other cases, the request or demand for assistance with a spiritual problem may arise when the nurse has no better resource than himself or herself. What does the nurse bring to this situation? In Chapter 7, we noted the nurse's lack of education in this area. Often the nurse may piece together what she knows about psychological counseling or psychiatric nursing along with what she knows from her own religious upbringing—if he or she had the latter experience. Immediately, we are thrown back into the question of levels—the nurse's and the patient's. In addition, we must worry about the match or mismatch.

DANGERS OF SPIRITUAL OR
RELIGIOUS INTERVENTIONS

When the nurse elects to treat a patient's spiritual issues, vulnerabilities appear. Some of the dangers of spiritual or religious interventions include:

1. Creating a situation where a less spiritually sophisticated nurse tries to counsel a more spiritually advanced patient
2. Forcing the nurse into a dual relationship with a patient (care provider and spiritual counselor)
3. Giving a nurse an opportunity for inappropriate proselytizing of his/her own religion
4. Allowing the nurse to usurp religious authority
5. Allowing the nurse to interrupt a patient's spiritual journey with false reassurances
6. Substituting health goals for spiritual goals
7. Assuming that all patients with the same spiritual nursing diagnosis need the same therapy
8. Assuming that all religious patients are the same and need the same spiritual therapy
9. Assuming that long-term therapies (e.g., meditation) can achieve spiritual goals in a short hospitalization time
10. Attempting to meld two visions of spirituality/religion (the nurse's and the patient's) that may be incompatible

Usually the patient interrupts the counseling when one of these failures occurs. Yet such a break can disrupt the regular caregiving relationship as well.

SPIRITUALITY AS A NURSING ELEMENT

If spirituality is a context of care, then what can be expected of nurses? It is illogical to reduce spirituality to cultural analysis (ritual aspects of religion). The first issue (as discussed in Chapter 1) is recognizing potential conflicts between spiritual goals and clinical care goals. As we have noted, most health care professionals simply assume that health care goals take precedence. However, some patients will be much more concerned with their spiritual goals. How does the nurse give credence to these patients' goal priorities?

It is important to see a way of supporting such a patient rather than attempting to change a patient's pathway to spiritual maturity. This may go against a nurses' desire to help or cure the disease/injury manifestations. It may be difficult for a nurse to see a patient struggle with spiritual issues, partly because spiritual struggles and spiritual pathways are not amenable to a quick fix. Yes, the nurse can be supportive, but no one can substitute their own spiritual journey for another person's journey. Nevertheless, some nurses will experience a need to cut short the patient's journey with facile reassurances.

At least some nursing groups have not wanted to give up the function of spiritual service—witness the spiritually related diagnoses in the North American Nursing Diagnosis Association (NANDA) documents (2009), the listing of spiritual competencies by the National Organization of Nurse Practitioner Faculties (NONPF) in (2002), or the spiritual items set by the Quality and Safety Education for Nurses Project (QSEN), in (2009). Although spirituality virtually disappeared when nursing was proving itself a valid academic discipline, it began in the last two decades to slip back into our focus. As these documents indicate, we find spiritual items not only reappearing but also being dictated for the practice world by accrediting and credentialing bodies.

How do nurses best handle spiritual matters that appear so often when patients face health care crises? Many patients' questions may invite the nurse to engage in a spiritual conversation. Alternately, many such questions, but not all of them, could be handled as psychological inquiries. What determines the nurse's choice? Usually, the nurse will sense when a psychological answer is avoiding what the patient is really asking. Moreover, if she/he offers mere shibboleths of reassurance, the nurse will know that is a matter of avoidance. Indeed, not all nurses are comfortable with spiritual questions.

Yet, ironically, others in the health care environment may be as unprepared as some nurses to deal with patients' spiritual challenges. We may even find the same unpreparedness in a chaplain or other religious leader. The answer for the nurse, to a great degree, will depend on his/her spiritual maturity. As we have seen, a person cannot respond on a higher level than that of his/her own personal achievement.

Remember, before the nurse acts in any way, she must know whether she is going to deal with health care objectives or spiritual objectives because these may be quite different. Indeed, they may even conflict with each other. As indicated in Chapter 4, often it is assumed that health care objectives will take precedence. Yet a patient may feel that spiritual objectives are more important. The nurse should recognize when he/she is selecting one sort of objective over another. This can be challenging if one is bound by objectives established by evaluating structures.

SPIRITUAL/RELIGIOUS THERAPIES

Sources list many alternative actions that the nurse might employ for a patient with a spiritual dilemma. Obviously, these methods would require matching to the patient's particular problems. Methods might include:

1. Prayer (by the patient, nurse, or other present person)
2. Intercessory prayer (by others known or unknown)
3. Forgiveness therapy (initiated by the patient or others)
4. Ritual behavior (e.g., use of rosary beads)
5. Psychological therapy (possibly spiritually oriented)
6. Relaxation therapy
7. Meditation
8. Use of religious contemplation or other visualization and guided imagery techniques
9. Reading a Bible or other guiding religious book
10. Development of a philosophy of religion or spirituality
11. Bibliotherapy (reading of related literature)
12. Discussion with religious leaders
13. Visits from one's religious community members
14. Confrontation therapy (including 12-Step programs with surrender to a Higher Power)
15. Exploring paths that offer hope or ways of coping
16. The patient experiencing the nurse or religious leader *being there*

SPIRITUAL/RELIGIOUS THERAPY: DECIDING WHAT WORKS

As Harris, Thoresen, McCullough, and Larson point out, many of these therapies could be offered as psychological assistance without a spiritual or religious context. This fact makes it challenging to associate many outcomes exclusively with spiritual or religious correlates. Hence, we have difficulty in knowing what therapies are truly spiritual. Further, as we noted in Chapter 5, spiritual and religious variables may be mixed in research tools, making it impossible to attribute results to one or another of these causes.

Another problem exists in that it is almost impossible to separate some of these methods for research purposes. For example, if intercessory prayers were the variable to be tested, there would be no way to stop others (e.g., family members) from also praying for the patient.

Larry Dossey's (1993) tests with people praying for various laboratory results (as opposed to praying for specific people) might be taken as one example designed to avoid the problem of being unable to isolate the variable of prayer. Yet in the clinical situation, the context makes it particularly difficult to determine what works and what doesn't.

Additionally, misapplication of some therapies may have negative results. For example, forgiveness therapy could prove disastrous if used for some patients. Suppose, for example, that one has a psychopathic patient who is unable to develop empathy for his victims. He may interpret forgiveness therapy as a license to continue his past victimizing behaviors.

SUMMARY

Providing spiritual care is not as simple as it appears. The nurse may face many challenges, including whether to even attempt it. Given their own belief systems, some nurses may not feel that they can ethically provide spiritual care. Others may have a real talent for it.

Logic dictates that nurses be able to provide (or not provide) spiritual care based on personal as well as professional attributes. Whatever their abilities, practicing nurses will be faced with spiritual issues, and should, at the very least, know in advance how they plan to manage such situations. In every case, the rights and beliefs of both patient and nurse need to be respected.

Sometimes a wide disparity can be bridged if the patient's queries can be handled as psychological inquiries. Statistics tell us that health care professionals are much less likely, for example, to believe in God than is the case with the public. It would not be wise for a nurse to promulgate this view when the patient is fixed on a spiritual journey. However it is managed, everyone's belief system should be handled with respect.

REFERENCE

Grosso, M. (Summer, 2009). What is spirituality? In *PsychoSpiritual Dialogue* (pp. 9–11). New York: Association for Spirituality and Psychotherapy.

BIBLIOGRAPHY

American Nurses' Association (2001). *Code of ethics with interpretive statement.* Washington, DC: Author.

Dossey, L. (1993). *Healing words.* San Francisco: HarperSanFrancisco.

Harris, A., Thoresen, C., McCullough, M., & Larson, D. (1999). Spirituality and religiously oriented health interventions. *Journal of Health Psychology, 4*(3), 413–433.

North American Nursing Diagnosis Association. (2009). *Nursing diagnoses: Definitions and classification 2009–2011.* In T. H. Herdman (Ed.). Hoboken, NJ: Wiley & Blackwell.

National Organization of Nurse Practitioner Faculties. (2002). *Domains and core competencies of nurse practitioner practice.* Washington, DC: Author.

Quality and Safety Education for Nurses Project. (2009). Patient-centered care, definition. *Nursing Outlook, 57*(6), 338–354.

CHAPTER 10

Today's Nursing: A Prisoner of Context?

The reader should be warned that this is a topic about which I hold a firm opinion. It won't take long for my bias to surface. Nor was I tempted to give the *other side* equal time. It is already winning the race for control of our profession.

Many chapters in this book have addressed (directly or indirectly) a major contextual dictate that holds us prisoner to one way of thinking today and one way of constructing our nursing education and practice plans. However, I haven't really called attention to it until this chapter. It is becoming a fact that in many settings, all our nursing actions are derived to meet preset outcome objectives: management objectives, clinical care objectives, case map objectives, and others. These objectives are helped along the way by various attempts to capture all our nursing diagnoses in a concrete and complete lexicon. However, for simplicity, I'm going to only label all these forms as outcome objectives.

These objectives seem like simple tools, but are they more powerful than we suspect? Do they control the whole environment in which nursing takes place? Moreover, how have we failed to recognize our bondage to this environment?

Equally important, how does that bondage hamper our work with spiritual aspects of care? And what would it mean to lift the bondage?

WHAT IS CONTEXT?

To understand the problem, first one has to have a good grasp of *context*. Indeed, the problem is all about context. All extant nursing practices and educational programs work from a theory of nursing. As we saw in Chapter 6, some of these theories are well spelled out. In other cases, some nurses may say that they work without a theory. Yet, if you examine the way they organize and distribute the work, you will find that the theory is present; it is just unstated. Indeed, if one watches a nursing unit long enough, one can identify the theory by which they are working.

Here is a simple example of just one theory element at work in a hospital unit. This element is delegation, an element that has changed over time. I'll begin with what was called *functional nursing*, a system that was historically once the norm. It was a theory under which I began my nursing career. In functional nursing, tasks were distributed among nurses according to the functions they performed. There was a medicine nurse, a treatment nurse, a bath-giving nurse, and so on. Supposedly, functional nursing was efficient. A nurse could become very skilled at a given task. It took a few decades for people to figure out that no matter how skilled the nurses are, none had a conception of the total patient.

Later this was changed to *team nursing*—where patients were distributed rather than tasks. A group of workers were assigned to a group of patients so that they could know them more intimately. Later that format was replaced by what was called *primary nursing*. Here the nurse had her own patients not just for a given day but for the length of their hospital stays. The attempt was to further hone what the nurse knew about her patients. The vulnerability in this system was that if a patient were assigned to an inexpert nurse, no one else was likely to notice the deficits in care that occurred.

In these three theories, the main factor (commonplace) is the work distribution. In observing actual work, one could identify other elements of theory organization. Part of each theory, for example, could be further defined by looking at how patients were distributed at admission. Were patients on a floor grouped by disease, by injury, or by therapy required?

Recognizing a theory in action is easier if one divides the elements into content, process, goal, and context. Mostly, these elements explain themselves. As a brief reminder, *content* is the subject matter. For example, in Newman's theory the subject matter, the main one, is *evolving consciousness*. *Process* refers to what the nurse does or thinks. It is the action element. *Goal* is the end point, the intended final result of applying the theory.

The element that is the most difficult to understand is *context*, which refers to the kind of world in which the given theory takes place. For example, in O'Brien's theory, the context is one where the patient is ill but focused on his or her spiritual well-being. The theory takes place only with patients having long-term illness, and the theory revolves around the spiritual or religious health of these patients. That is the world (context) in which O'Brien's patients find themselves.

Because recognizing the context of a theory is the most difficult part of understanding a theory, nurses are often unaware of the nature of the context in which they are working. The easiest way to explain this is to think of a fish being unaware that his context is water—until he is hauled out of it.

Yet context is very important to any practice. At present, one of the most important elements of the practice and education of nurses is the *context* created by outcome objectives. And many nurses fail to understand the way in which outcome objectives become part of the context. True, outcome objectives are also goals, but their dominance over the work design changes the way nurses think about their work. Sometimes this happens by choice but more often because accrediting and evaluating bodies require objectives.

Remember Margaret Newman protesting against reductive theories (Chapter 6). For her theory to work, the nurse must give up her control of outcomes. The patient's process of evolving consciousness must go wherever it goes. It may, indeed, reach levels of expansion that the nurse never imagined in her wildest dreams. That is the joy of Newman's theory. Notice what a different environment this is from the one where nurses are programmed to think in terms of preset objectives.

It is also the reason one will seldom see Newman's theory used today. Where accrediting agencies hold power, her theory simply could not be instituted, at least not as Newman envisioned it. At present, virtually all our accrediting agencies require that outcome objectives be set in advance and thereafter be used as criteria for judging the effectiveness of the program.

This is a great requirement for accreditors because it gives them clear criteria for their evaluations. Either the organization has reached, or failed to reach, its own outcome objectives. What could be fairer? However, such a system wouldn't work for a Newman-dominated education or practice. Open-ended goals? Impossible! Yet it is not just Newman's theory of nursing that is impaled on the tyranny of the outcome objective. Martha Rogers's theory, for example, would fare no better. Many other nursing theories and other practices also could be discriminated against. Programs forced to implement outcome objectives necessarily use them to organize the work.

TRAPPED IN WILBER'S UPPER RIGHT HAND QUADRANT

The use of outcome objectives has several strikes against it. The first issue is one of location, and that can be best understood by going back to Wilber's "Four Quadrants of the Kosmos" (Chapter 5). Because outcome objectives tend to be written in specific operationalized format (for easy evaluation), they are written in the third-person, objective quadrant. In other words, they tend to occur in Wilber's upper right quadrant.

This is the quadrant that is labeled the *it* quadrant, where the elements are separate from the researcher or evaluator. Looking at organisms under a microscope is a good example. Objectives here are very formulaic. They come with no ambiguity, and anyone can evaluate their achievement. In essence, the evaluator does not influence the judgment. Theoretically, any evaluator will come away with the same conclusions. Quite simply, in terms of Wilber's four quadrants, these outcome objectives would fit in the upper right hand quadrant, the quadrant that is the so-called third-person *objective* one.

The method of thought in this upper right hand quadrant tends to be logistic (and reductive). Logistic thought explains a thing by reference to its parts, that is, *reducing* it to smaller pieces. For this upper right hand quadrant, reductive thinking feels like the essence of logic.

Now we are ready to look at the theories that best represent Wilber's upper right hand quadrant. The reader will recall that there was an historical era when it was asserted that *only* this quadrant was *scientific*, and that belief was labeled *Logical Positivism* (Chapter 5). This is when Freud tried to prove himself a proper scientist by fitting his theories into this philosophy, in other words into the upper right hand quadrant. However, he wasn't very successful once people recognized the difference between material and conceptual entities. Superego, id, and ego did not convert to this view of reality. These elements could not be found apart from the person using them. They were a conceptual system not a matter of material existence. Freud's system was shifted to where it belonged, into the *upper left hand quadrant*.

About this time, people recognized that research was not limited to the upper right quadrant but that every quadrant has its own proper forms of research. This is not to say that the upper right hand placement is a bad quadrant. Indeed, modern medicine wouldn't be where it is today but for this quadrant. My objection is not to the quadrant; my objection occurs when this is taken as the only quadrant, with attempts to mold all content to fit into it.

Accepting Logical Positivism was nursing's first context error, but it wasn't the last one. We also spent time arguing about holistic nursing care versus traditional care, that is, upper left hand care versus an upper right hand orientation. We finally learned that they could coexist without the world falling apart. Now, once again, the same argument is happening under current context control through the device of outcome objectives.

We seem to be vulnerable to one-quadrant-fits-all thinking. In addition to the initial arguments against holistic nursing, we also saw a great struggle between two advanced practice models: the clinical nurse specialist and the nurse practitioner. Here we faced the same quadrant issues, with the greatest professional resistance against the nurse practitioner role. When nurse practitioner programs began, most of them were originally taught by physicians who used the methods they knew best (upper right hand quadrant, logistic). These practitioner ideologies were cast against their opposite number, more traditional nursing specialist curricula, which were typically a mix, with much content from the upper left hand quadrant. The nurse practitioner role and the clinical specialist role were seen as two different methods for approaching nursing.

Just as happened in Logical Positivism, there was an era of competition. Indeed, some of our most famous nurse theorists took the position that nurse practitioners weren't even nurses. Not surprisingly, Martha Rogers was chief among them. Similar to Newman, Roger's own theory was located in the upper left hand quadrant. And that's why she felt that the practitioner programs were a threat.

However, eventually nurses learned that these two camps, these two ways of thinking, could live with each other quite successfully. There was no need to tear down one system to validate the other.

Ironically, our adoption of outcome objectives threatens to take us back to these historical either/or mistakes, without ever saying a word about what is happening. Once again this tactic sets one quadrant against the others. We face a challenge that demands we put all our theories in the same basket. This time, it is the third-person, upper right hand quadrant that is taking over as the only view of the world, the only form of thinking that counts.

Notice that, if the nurse, the director of a school, or the vice president of nursing practice *must* construct his or her systems to comply with the outcome objectives format, he or she has effectively been stopped from using the other quadrants. Yet, because it isn't given a label this time, we fail to recognize that this compulsory practice is happening. In addition, we have succumbed to the tyranny of the upper right hand quadrant of Wilber's metatheory: the tyranny of the outcome objective.

Because this new tyranny is through *context*, the least visible aspect of theory, many of us don't even understand that we are being held prisoner by this format.

PAST, PRESENT, AND FUTURE

It is a great limitation on nursing when we accept that there is only *one right way* of doing things. It is the virtual end of vision, and that is a very strong manacle. Outcome objectives, clinical care by objectives, case management protocols, care maps, and management by objectives are notions that limit nursing to the already known, the already tested, and the findings of the present or past eras. This is inevitable because outcome objectives come from the past. They do not represent a vision from the future.

In this context, for example, it would be nonsense to set an object for greater or quicker recovery than the norm. There would be no nurse thinking, *I bet we could achieve more for this particular patient if we do this instead.* There is no encouragement for that sort of thinking. As Newman might say, we have lost our ability to dream of a future.

Outcome objectives give us clinical care maps with preset objectives for patients of every diagnosis, with every impairment or every surgery. Everything is nicely spelled out. Sometimes objectives are reworded as competencies—but the construct is the same. Notice what a secure world this creates: Everything is known, the nurse can't make a mistake if he or she follows the formula. Moreover, frankly, there's not much reason for him or her to think about it. The patient with a different level of motivation or the patient who may not want to conform to our preset objectives will not have different objectives.

We like objectives, and they give us clear directions. We can spell them out in clear unambiguous terms and in clearly demarcated options. There's just one problem with objectives—well, at least one problem: Objectives assume that we already have the answers. Objectives *are* answers. So if someone happens to contrast objectives with, let's say, vision, then vision has to go. Vision looks toward answers yet to be found, toward things that may come into being in the future. Vision looks to domains not yet chopped up and divided among objectives.

With our fixation on objectives, nursing becomes a profession in search of finite answers, finite security, and a checklist by which to know that we did the right thing. That's okay for many subject matters but not for everything. Some things can be managed that way—the length of time one is contagious after a given infection and the way a given procedure can be administered with safety. However, new possibilities disappear when we think we already have all the answers.

CREATIVITY AND VISION

Creativity and vision have to do with the future in the sense that they deal with the new, the unknown, and the untested. They can't occur under the dictate that we follow the established rules, with the answers already laid out in given objectives. In other words, if we are forced to use a system created in the past and/or present, we never look to the future.

We are brought back to Newman's notion that the nurse cannot know the final answers. In today's context, we are often restricted by what we already know, dedicated to the objectives we have already conceived. Under this model, nursing becomes very much like a car assembly line: We know the pieces and what product we'll have if we put them together in the correct order. Yes, we'll have very well operating cars—but they will be very similar cars.

In many cases, the car assembly line is enough but not in all matters. Some maverick nurses may be bored to death on assembly line nursing. Moreover, these mavericks are often the ones who bring about new paradigms, new thoughts, and new imagination in patient care. Do we really want to bore them out of the profession?

CONTEXT VERSUS SPIRITUALITY

Being imprisoned in the upper right hand quadrant is very important when we are considering theories that take spirituality into account, simply because spiritual values usually appear in Wilber's upper *left* hand quadrant—which means that they work on different rules. They aren't characterized by concreteness but by their conceptual nature.

Spirituality by its nature is distorted if it is shifted to the right hand (objective) side of Wilber's map of reality. Recall what lengths Fowler went to in order to create detailed verbal descriptions of the different levels of spirituality that occurred on the left hand side. Yet is spirituality an illusion because it can't be measured with a ruler? Is it an illusion because it can vary from one person to the next? Things in the upper left hand quadrant deal with subtle and complex concepts. The upper right hand quadrant couldn't tolerate such ambiguity.

What happens is that the essence of spirituality (if shifted to the upper right hand quadrant) is vulnerable to being lost in the domain of objective concreteness. Spirituality belongs in the left hand upper quadrant of *me* as Dossey and Newman correctly realized.

When we insist that spirituality fit the context of Wilber's upper right quadrant, it disappears, and this is ironic in a profession that once claimed that its roots lay in spirituality or religion. Religion, depending on how it is conceived, may suffer from the same fate. On the other hand, it has enough definable variables (e.g., attendance at church, frequency of prayer, and amount of fiscal contributions) to adapt to some types of operationalized objectives.

Spirituality, alas, has few universal variables. Spirituality was consumed in the *art* of nursing, when nursing was called an art and a science. The new student, however, will hear little about these roots. In truth, the student is likely to hear little about the origins of the profession—perhaps a few references to Florence Nightingale as if nursing began with her. It is typical that today Nightingale is praised as a scientist, an environmentalist, and a statistician. This is not to say that these things were not true about her within the constraints of the knowledge of her era. However, almost nothing will be heard about the fact that she also listened to a mystical *voice* and spent much of her life fluctuating between the pulls of the Anglican and Catholic churches.

Clearly, if one roots professional nursing in Nightingale, as is usually done, one should recognize that nursing developed as a tension between the spirit and science of nursing. At one time, nursing was content to give equal credit to these two polarities. However, that ended when nursing sought its place in academe. The die was cast in favor of the scientific end of the continuum. Perhaps we could have predicted the coming slippage into the present world of everything being managed by outcome objectives.

Ironically, it is probably still the case that the majority of students enter nursing with intentions that might best be called spiritual rather than scientific. Few students verbalize a desire to work in a science when entering the school, although faculty immediately begin to indoctrinate them in that heritage rather than building on their spiritual yearnings to care for the sick.

It is not fair to say that one quadrant (upper right) favors science and another (upper left) does not. Each quadrant has its own fitting forms of science. Otherwise, we would not have such masterful left hand tools as Fowler's, Piaget's, Erickson's, and Maslow's stages of development. These deal with conceptual systems and not with matters of objective fact of the type handled in the right hand quadrant.

My objection to a context set by outcome objectives, then, is that it wants to see *all* of nursing through a single eye—the so-called scientific viewpoint of the upper right hand quadrant. There is little tolerance for anyone who wants to view nursing through a different lens. My next objection is that this format is impenetrable to spiritual virtues. Spiritual values don't fit in this quadrant any more than did Freud's id, ego, and superego.

What I want to do in this next section is give the reader a sense of what would happen to a spiritual philosophy when it hits the wall created by outcome objectives. Take, for example, Jon Kabat-Zinn (1994):

> . . . Inquiry is not just a way to solve problems. It is a way to make sure you are staying in touch with the basic mystery of life itself and of our presence here . . . Inquiry doesn't mean looking for answers, especially quick answers which come out of superficial thinking. It means asking without expecting answers, just pondering the question, carrying the wondering with you, letting it percolate, bubble, cook, ripen, come in and out of awareness, just as everything else comes in and out of awareness. (p. 233)

How, indeed, is an accrediting agency going to judge if patients are *staying in touch with the basic mystery of life*? Okay, if you want spirituality in your nursing theories, make up an outcome objective for that. While you're doing it, keep in mind that the objective can't lose any of the meaning, the emotion, and the intensity. Remember, you can't capture Edgar Allan Poe's *The Raven* with an objective such as *Writes about large black birds with negative attitudes*. It loses something in the translation.

Or take James Hillman (1996):

> Invisibility perplexes the American common sense and American psychology which hold as a major governing principle that whatever exists, exists in some quantity and therefore can be measured. If an image in the heart that calls you to your fate exists, and may be strong and long-lasting, has it measurable dimensions? A passion to cage the invisible by visible methods continues to motivate the science of psychology, even though that science has given up the century-long search for the soul in various body parts and systems. (p. 92)

I don't need to tell you what Hillman would think of the outcome objective if you can read the paragraph above. That is, unless you can think of a system of spirituality without a soul.

Or look at what Deepak Chopra (2000) says:

> Reality is constantly flowing from the virtual level to the quantum to the material. In mystical terms, this constant movement is called "the river of life," because to the mystic everything begins in the mind of God before it appears on the surface as an event or object. But the river is more than a metaphor. With every thought, memory, and desire, we take a journey upriver, from our invisible source to our material destinations. (pp. 211–212)

A system of outcome objectives would have difficulty with a movement that starts in the invisible. Are you beginning to see why the spiritual can't bow to an outcome objective?

As one more example, let's take M. Scott Peck (1997):

> And to our limited vision God is inevitably mysterious. Since our souls are ongoing creations of God, through them we partake in God and thereby, whether we like it or not, we partake in His mystery. (pp. 157–158)

Again, we have spiritual ideas that escape outcome objectives. Nor can we say that meeting spiritual needs is a part of nursing and then put in place a system that, by its very nature, cannot deal with spirituality.

SUMMARY

I find a major conflict between most notions of spirituality and the context of our typical operationalized outcome objectives. Other quadrants have their own evaluation formats, albeit in different forms. Perhaps we might need to decide which way we're going. Or are we incapable of recognizing incompatibilities? Or, radically, could we admit that not all our work can be submitted to concrete outcome objectives? Why can't we just leave things in the quadrant where they fit?

So that's the end of my plea that we let at least some of our members and some of our ideas escape from the context that threatens to absorb the whole nursing world. Yes, it's orderly. But must we all march to the same drummer? Yes, it's a drummer (outcome objectives) that can achieve many good things. However, they must be the right things, the things that fit with outcome objectives. In addition, these objectives are a drummer that will never envision things that fall outside of the upper right hand quadrant. Yes, it's a box that can be modified when things happen. Patients start waking up from prolonged comas—something that is new on the scene. Therefore, we may add an objective that makes us take better care against contractures—just in case. However, is that as creative as we want to be? Or reactive creativity?

We have all met patients who we *know* will exceed our preplanned objectives. We know it because we sense something mysterious about their souls. What should we do with such maverick patients? Dare we handle them differently? If nothing else, what might we learn from them? Or do we just say, *well that patient isn't in spiritual distress and that's our objective. So we'll just pass him by.* Is that the world of nursing that we want? (I won't even go into the arrogance assumed when we think we can relieve a patient's spiritual distress.)

I'm afraid of where we may take the profession when we deal only with aspects of certainty, with norms, and with the already known. Must we worship at the upper right quadrant? What will this model do to those nurses who want their care to include spiritual dialog? Will it still our voices? Will it contract our minds? Will it make the spiritual so superficial that we should give up on it?

Alternatively, are we capable of seeing both the virtues and the limitations of preset concrete outcome objectives? Are we able to recognize how they can take over and control the nature of our practice? Can we understand how they structure our environment?

REFERENCES

Chopra, D. (2000). *How to know God: The soul's journey into the mystery of mysteries.* New York: Harmony Books.

Hillman, J. (1996). *The soul's code: In search of character and calling.* New York: Warner Books.

Kabat-Zinn, J. (1994). *Wherever you go there you are.* New York: Hyperion.

Peck, M. S. (1997). *Denial of the soul.* New York: Harmony Books.

CHAPTER 11

Dying, Death, Disability, and Despair

It's impossible to write a book on spirituality without considering patients in the most extreme conditions. These people are those most likely to be experiencing or seeking spiritual states. I've elected to look at patients facing dying, death, disability, and/or despair. Here, I'm thinking of patients for whom medicine had played its part and has little left to contribute. These patients often are in states where spiritual efforts may be the only remaining open gate.

Dying and *death* inspire fear, resignation, lack of resignation, rage, and/or acceptance, among other emotional states. Unless a patient is unconscious or unaware of his or her situation, this transition invariably raises emotions, and a review of spiritual beliefs and hopes usually plays a part. When I speak of *disability* in this chapter, I am only considering the most extreme impairments, those from which one can expect little improvement, dire disabilities that change a life pattern just for survival.

Despair, unlike the preceding terms, is an emotion, a feeling, whereas dying, death, and disability refer to physical states of being, albeit they are states likely to evoke emotional responses. Despair can and often does, attach to these states. By despair, I don't mean depression. I mean the deepest sort of soul rending, where the patient is bereft of everything one needs to face a burden and carry on a life.

What happens from a spiritual perspective when a person faces the most extreme life situations? In what way does spirituality contribute in such situations? Are these exactly the situations that may turn a person toward the spiritual? What can or should the nurse do for such a patient? What does the nurse do when the desire to help may interfere with a patient's need to struggle toward a higher spiritual state?

BLAME

When we speak of states of dying, death, and disability, one thing that often is attached to them is blame. The disabled feel the brunt of judgment more often than the others in our society.

Blame is a great horror that can occur to people in dire and desperate states. And that occurs when someone else, or the person himself or herself, feels that he or she is responsible for what happened or is happening to him or her. Unfortunately, a lot of this blaming goes on. Ironically, some newer ideas seem to ratify that position if they are considered superficially: *You create your own reality. You invoke karma for past bad deeds.* These and other slogans can lead to placing blame on the already suffering victim.

When it comes to blame, I have learned the most about it through a technique I use with psychotherapy patients: past life regression. Unfortunately, the only way I can link these two notions incurs a brief *aside* here. Psychiatric nurses may recall that Freud originally used hypnosis with his patients. And that's the technique that has enhanced many of my perceptions including greater understanding of the topics in this chapter.

Freud said that he quit using hypnosis on his patients because he wasn't very good at it. But I suspect that Freud wasn't the type to admit he was ineffective at anything. My own suspicion is that he may have found himself acquiring information from patients that conflicted with his atheist beliefs, and that the easiest way to deal with that contradiction was to simply cut out the source. The methods that he substituted guaranteed that the patient's thoughts would stay within the present lifetime.

Let me say first, that *past life regression* is an inaccurate term because clients can also go to future lives (*progression* instead of regression) or to existence between lives. But for simplicity, I'll term all these altered states simply as regression. Hypnosis is not the only way to reach these states, but it is the simplest. Regression may also lead to very early but suppressed parts of the present life. For example, I've had many clients track a psychological problem to things that have happened to them in the first year of life, even during their births.

About 90% of my clients seek regression because of psychological problems. The remaining clients are simply interested in experiencing these altered states. Of the clients seeking to resolve psychological problems, a large number are referred by psychiatrists or analysts who have been unable to find causation for problems in the patient's present life. Most of these clients (and their therapists) seek answers to psychological problems in past lives, so I'll mostly speak of that state.

In my use of past life regression, I've found sources of severe disabilities, instances of what seem to be premature death of significant others, or particularly difficult paths of dying. Use of past life regression implies the reality of a few other principles, among them, reincarnation. Although this is the easiest explanation for what clients discover when they find themselves in different bodies and different eras, it is not the only possible explanation. Indeed, I think it is likely that more than one source of past lives may be in play.

However, I believe that the past lives that a client recounts are important regardless of whether they actually occurred to that person in a past life. Wherever they come from, the past lives inevitably give clues to the client's present problems. Pragmatically, I don't particularly care if the past lives were *real* or come from some other source. The important thing is that they are helpful to the client.

Another principle associated with past lives is that the lives people lead here (and elsewhere) appear to be purposeful learning situations. As we found in levels of spirituality (Chapter 5), there seem to be people at different levels of learning. I find this principle intertwined with the notion of reincarnation in clients' reports. In regression, it is very common for people to perceive various lives as cumulative lessons. And there is usually agreement that any earth life is one of the more difficult choices. Once clients have started reincarnating on earth, it is likely that they will have a series of lives here.

This, of course, implies that there are other options, many of which are reported by clients. So perhaps, a third principle is that reality has many more choices for exploration beyond our single planet circulating around a slowly dying sun.

The reader who wishes to say hogwash to the notions of reincarnation, continuous learning, and a very complex and expanded notion of reality may simply want to skip this chapter because these notions certainly influence my ideas of reality.

Having said that, I find the following reasons for turning a skeptical eye on blame. First, during regression, I hear from many clients that they (or a significant other) have chosen a life or a portion of a life with severe disability or early death as a learning experience or to assist someone else with a learning experience.

Interestingly, I also find two contrasting temperaments among people: first, those who want to learn the slow and easy way, with more lives but having less difficult lessons in any one life. Their opposites prefer more difficult (but fewer) lives for quicker learning. Included in the latter group might be people who elect the experience of extreme disability or early death.

Other people may elect a disabled body as the only choice available to put them in a situation where they wish to be. Others, indeed, might choose a disabled and difficult life as a karmic lesson. At no time have I ever heard a client say that he/she was being punished by some higher level judgment.

Learning occurs; punishment does not—unless the person inflicts it on himself or herself.

In a related pattern, some clients ask questions such as *Things come to me with such difficulty. How is it that everything comes so easily to my sister?* In regression, some clients find that the sister, wife, husband, or other is on what I label a *vacation life* after having experienced a series of difficult lives.

Alternately, many disabled clients claim that there truly are unplanned accidents on this planet. Not everything that happens is programmed in advance. So an accidental injury might simply be that: an accident.

Additionally, in regression there is much agreement that everyone finds at least one personal guide on a spiritual level. Some people claim that their guides are responsible to some extent for their education in this school called Earth. Some claim that, if they don't learn a lesson the easy way, the guide may send a more challenging situation to impress the lesson to be learned.

This claim makes me recall an incident I observed between a lawyer acquaintance and his wife. They were a couple in their early 60s who had inherited the task of raising their two young grandchildren, one of whom was both physically and mentally challenged. This child received a lot of special care from a physical therapist and a speech therapist.

I was once sitting beside the wife at a small dinner party during the holidays. The wife, who might seem a bit old fashioned to most of us, leaned over the table and asked her husband for some extra money because she wanted to buy gifts for the little girl's two therapists.

The lawyer husband answered bluntly, "Absolutely not. They picked low paying jobs; it was their choice—they could have studied for better paying careers if they had the motivation." The wife simply accepted this judgment. But I remember feeling a chill run down my spine, a sense of dread when he made that speech.

Four months later, the husband suffered a paralyzing injury while skiing. He was hospitalized for many months, followed by many months of rehabilitation that, for much of the first year, left him without control of bodily functions and unable to walk. After much rehabilitation, he regained bodily control and learned to walk with a walker. When I visited him in the hospital about a month after his initial injury, he told me that whether his days were good or bad totally depended on how things went that day with his physical therapist.

He said this with no particular insight, but my mind immediately went back to that evening at the dinner table. Was his guide simply giving him a harder lesson because he had failed to get the earlier message? I have no idea, but I couldn't help wondering.

In any case, I've never found a client claim that a difficult or disabled life was a matter deserving of blame. Most blame comes from the client himself.

Yet our society produces many people willing to place blame and judgment on others. Unfortunately, some of these judgmental people are health care workers. My practice has continually reinforced the notion that things are much more complicated than such a narrow interpretation implies. Blame is never a productive path.

DYING AND DEATH

Elisabeth Kubler-Ross, MD (1969, 1975), brought to a crashing end the social silence concerning death and dying when she identified the final stages of dying: denial, rage and anger, bargaining, depression, and acceptance (1975). Every one of these stages may push patients into various spiritual states for both good and ill.

Kubler-Ross' findings ushered in a whole new era of honesty in informing patients and their families about incipient death. Although some people still show an old-fashioned recalcitrance in dealing with death, many now are able to deal with it forthrightly.

Although her work has acceptance now, I was at the University of Chicago Hospitals and Clinics when she was working with dying patients there. She found herself greatly stigmatized by the medical staff at that time. She did not have an easy career among her physician peers for many years.

Further, in later years her reputation was not enhanced when she became interested in various paranormal phenomena. The reader can decide whether her interests were appropriate by reading her (1997) book *The wheel of life: A memoir of living and dying*. But whatever the diagnosis on this issue, it can't detract from the strength of her work on the stages of dying.

Ironically, Kubler-Ross's work was accepted much earlier in nursing than in her own discipline of medicine. I think that the psychologies of the two fields have much to do with this. For many physicians, there is no such thing as a *good death*; death is cast as the enemy. Yet, nurses can immediately determine whether a patient had a good or bad death. The criterion isn't the *fact* of death but the very human context in which the death occurs.

HOSPICE

The hospice movement was the first significant mass movement to deal with the issue of dying from a philosophic perspective, enabling many people to die at home in dignity or in institutions whose philosophy accepted the inevitability of approaching deaths. This philosophy still allows people to avoid the often torturous end-of-life processes that so often occur in a hospital institution.

Hospice care also counteracts the all too human pattern (by both staff and family) of deserting of the dying. In our society, many people still respond to approaching death by avoidance. Many feel discomfort in being with a dying person. Denial is another common defense, one that often leaves a dying person unable to discuss the situation with others. How often have nurses heard, "Don't be silly, Daddy. Of course, you're not dying." This attitude is changing with more people accepting death as a socially acceptable topic of discussion. Nevertheless, many dying people still suffer the social imposition of a gag order by those who can only deal with death through denial.

PREDEATH PHENOMENA

Two types of unusual encounters occur to patients who are nearing death. NDEs and *predeath experiences*. NDEs occur when a person is pronounced dead and then is resuscitated. These encounters are reviewed in Chapter 3. From a spiritual perspective, the most important problem in both kinds of experiences may be a conflict between health care professionals wishing to discount these visions and patients who find them to be totally real and often life changing. Here's a partial report from one of Melvin Morse's (1990) patients. When this patient was in the midst of her NDE and resistant to returning to life, she was given the following vision. We might call this a vision within a vision. The patient said:

> I saw a tall blond man walking with two children. The little girl jumped up and down and her curls shook. The other was a boy. I recognized this as being my future family. I felt a longing for my husband and children even before I had met them. (p. 123)

The sense of reality in this NDE was reinforced when the same people appeared in her subsequent life.

The second type of encounter is the *predeath* experience. Predeath is the label that has been given to phenomena in which the dying (but not yet deceased) person sees visions, usually of deceased relatives, but sometimes of angels or religious figures. The visits usually occur in the last weeks or days of life, most commonly just a few days or hours before death. Sometimes the visitors tell patients that they will be accompanying them. These visions can offer great spiritual comfort to many patients.

Here Morse (1994) reports a vision of a child with leukemia as reported by her mother:

> I asked her what she saw, and she said that there was a boy at the end of the bed. . . . Over the next couple of days she carried on conversations with him and was glad to have him there. With everything that was going on, it was almost as though this little boy that only she could see was stability for her. I think he was an angel. (pp. 16–17)

A few other phenomena occur at the final predeath time. First, immediately before death, many patients who have been comatose or confused may suddenly have a moment of clarity and speak normally to those around them. Indeed, nurses used to caring for dying patients are likely to recognize this pattern of sudden clarity as indicating the immediate period before death.

Another common predeath event occurs when patients report seeing scenes or deceased visitors at about three feet off the floor. This may occur at death or periodically for months or weeks before the death. Some people infer from this that the next *level* of reality exists in vibrations that occur at that level relative to Earth. Whatever the reason, it is interesting that many people report this predeath phenomenon, even when they may have total clarity except for these episodic visions. Often, these visions have no particular message. It is as if the person just suddenly glanced through a different window—perhaps a preview of coming attractions.

There has always been a subtle contest between spirituality and death. One would say that truly spiritual persons who believe in a continued existence, albeit in a different form, should be comfortable with the concept of death. Yet, at least in our society, most people have a dread of death and try to postpone it if possible. Unless pain and suffering make death look better, most people still fear the transition to an unknown state. Persons who have had previous NDEs just don't fear death.

MANAGING GRIEF AFTER A DEATH

On a different issue, some people have great difficulty managing grief when a significant other dies. Psychiatrists sometimes refer patients to me who have become stuck in the grieving process. Somehow, these patients have convinced themselves (consciously or unconsciously) that continued grieving is the only way to honor the deceased. Often, this pattern can be stopped by having the client experience a past or future life with the person who has died. Because people tend to reincarnate in familiar groups, the client can often find other lives with the deceased and be reassured that they will likely meet again in future lives.

Alternately, some clients can simply be introduced to the concept that prolonged grieving is thought to burden the deceased by tying them to Earth. I recall one patient for whom just this altered notion of grieving was all she needed to hear. It had never occurred to her that grieving could be a hindrance rather than an honor to her mother. After 3 prior years of intractable grieving, she threw her mother a *bon voyage* party with all her old friends invited. She sent her mother on her way, toasting with champagne and releasing an array of balloons. That was the end of the client's grieving.

DISABILITY

Most nurses who care for patients with severe disabilities can recount tales of some patients who were truly inspirational and others who never got over despair or anger. The ones who were able to rise above major disabilities are usually those who hold strong spiritual beliefs. Such human abilities show a valor that has much to do with long lifetime patterns integrated into the patient's being. These patterns may reflect a particular spiritual or religious belief structure or not.

One thinks of amazing exemplars such as Steven Hawking, the British theoretical physicist who has lived a renowned life despite almost total body paralysis due to amyotrophic lateral sclerosis. Lay people know his work through his popular best seller, *A Brief History of Time* (1990). Why are some people capable of rising above extreme circumstance when others are not? There is no simple answer to that question, no one-size-fits-all response.

In the case of Hawking, it is evident that he has at least one compensation: A marvelous brain that was still able to keep in contact with the world. In reality, not all patients have such a release. In the next section on despair, we will see that death is not always the hardest path. Being severely disabled and unable to die may be much more horrible for the mind.

In this chapter, I want to illustrate the benefit of having a middle-range theory to assist in determining nursing care, in this case, care for the disabled. The reader who wants the full details of this theory can consult Florence Selder's (1982, 1989) works on *Life Transition Theory*. In personal correspondence, Dr. F. E. Selder, RN, PhD (2010), describes the theory in the following way, using as example a disability caused by spinal cord injury:

> Life Transition Theory (LTT) is one way to understand spirituality from a nursing perspective. The transition permits the person to become aware that life is permanently and irreversibly altered.

LTT is about the restructuring of a personal reality after a life-altering decision or a disruptive crucial event. A transition occurs when neither the decision nor the disrupting event can be integrated into the existing reality. It makes sense that, if a reality is disrupted, then one's point of view, values, beliefs, and sense of self (among other things) must be reconsidered. A person with a spinal cord injury cannot live as if he or she were able-bodied. If the patient attempts to live as able bodied, then rehabilitation could be compromised. Uncertainty marks this part of the transition

Uncertainty is part of any life transition. Uncertainty is a form of suffering, and a nurse uses strategies that reduce that uncertainty. For some patients, uncertainty can be cast within a spiritual framework. Nursing responses include giving information and providing resources. A nurse knows that simply being in a transition for a period of time helps the person to become less uncertain. Thus, the nurse lends support by giving time and his or her presence.

Knowing that the nurse will be there as the person recovers from the injury reduces uncertainty. It assures him or her that he or she is not alone. The nurse must be conscious of his or her role in being a presence for the person as a way of creating an intervention. Routine and unreflective nursing care does not create the space for the resolution of uncertainty and can increase suffering.

The transition itself reduces uncertainty as the person becomes aware of their changed circumstances through a series of *trigger events*. Two trigger events will be described, as well as how a nurse can facilitate the patient moving through the transition. The nurse can anticipate trigger events and frame the experiences as facilitating a person's progress through the transition. *Reactivation* is a trigger event that not only is a remembering of thoughts but also an experiencing of feelings and sensations that center on the decision or the disrupting event. It is easy for the person to feel off-balance when reactivation happens. For instance, a mother sobs when she hears tires screeching in a mall parking lot as it reminds her of her young daughter's death.

The nurse can reassure a patient that reactivation is normal and will diminish over time. Reactivation can also bring solace as this process shifts from centering on the disruption reality to being a source of comfort. One mother reported that twenty years after her daughter's death, she found her fur coat in the attic and it still had the daughter's perfume along with fine blond hairs on it. She held the coat and it felt as if she was holding her daughter. Knowledge about how to use reactivation, a natural occurring experience in a transition, fosters the person's strengths instead of deficits.

Irrevocability is a trigger event that brings about the awareness of the irreversibility of the changed reality. The nurse can be excited about a person with a spinal cord injury getting into a wheelchair for the first time. From the person's perspective getting into a wheelchair for the first time means, as one person said, "This is it, this is how my life will be." If the nurse fails to recognize that some markers of progress are also a source of suffering, then she misses an opportunity to help the patient through his transition.

In addition to becoming aware that one's reality must change, a person is faced with containing the intrusiveness of the event (disease, spinal cord injury) or decision (to divorce, undergo therapy). Living with a chronic disease, disability, or a loss such as a death of a child or the inability to have a baby brings about spiritual challenges. While the patient is undergoing the transition to a new reality, he or she may be undergoing a spiritual transition as well.

Concurrent with the emergence of a new reality is the *meaning-making* that occurs with *restructuring*. The processes that occur with containing intrusion are less important in the realm of spirituality than the ideal of helping persons make meaning of what has happened to them. Novice nurses are tempted to give platitudes, reassurances, and advice as a way to help persons find meaning in what has happened to them. The expert nurse knows that meaning making is a complex process including listening to the subtext of the patient's words and providing an environment for the person's reflection.

The process of meaning-making is lengthy, and the nurse may facilitate the process at various times during the process. It is likely the nurse will work with some persons who are not finding meaning in what has happened to them. Some call this a spiritual crisis. The nurse must hold the potential reality for the person, a reality that can be satisfying and meaningful.

The most challenging actions for the nurse are to know himself or herself and to use reflection as one works with the person. If the nurse cannot see a meaningful future for the people he or she works with, then it will be more difficult for them. A man with a spinal injury, who earlier reported that the injury had made his life better, subsequently told the nurse that he wasn't sure that he would make it. He had found out that the police car (without sirens) that went through a red light and hit his car, had not been going anywhere. At that point, the man had no meaning for what had happened to him. As long as he thought the police were speeding to help someone else, his injury had meaning.

In summary, the beginning of the transition is about becoming aware of the permanently changed situation leading to the transition. The nurse can use knowledge of transition theory in his or her work with patients and in helping them to resolve their spiritual crises. The nurse does this by reducing uncertainty and lessening the intrusions on the disrupted reality. Making sense or making meaning of what has happened is an essential part of the transition.

In this way, the nurse has a structure to approach the patient with a severe disability. The same information applies to nursing a person who has sustained a death of a significant other. Selder's theory is useful in many extreme cases of life transition.

DESPAIR

As we indicated earlier, despair is an emotion that may occur in dying or disability (among other circumstances). The philosopher Soren Kierkegaard (1954) called despair *the Sickness Unto Death* (p. 150).

So to be sick unto death is, not to be able to die—yet not as though there were hope of life; no, the hopelessness in this case is that even the last hope, death, is not available. (pp. 150–151)

So when the danger is so great that death has become one's hope, despair is the disconsolateness of not being able to die. (p. 151)

Kierkegaard's work, a classic on despair, provides a description that enables one to differentiate it from a more simple form of depression. Coming from a religious orientation, Kierkegaard notes that ". . . the majority of men live without being thoroughly conscious that they are spiritual beings . . ." (p. 159)

Nurses often identify helping the patient *cope* as a spiritual therapy. Coping ability is what patients in despair lack. But helping patients build coping strategies is a useful therapy where a patient is able to benefit from it. Coping, or the attempt to cope, is a positive sign that one is leaving despair and embracing hope.

Beginning in Chapter 1, we noticed that nursing objectives and spiritual objectives may clash with each other. The nurse's desire to *help* may take the form of encouraging the patient to regress spirituality to a prior more comfortable form of religion or spirituality. Nurses sometimes do this because they have difficulty observing a patient struggle with spiritual challenges. If the nurse is working with nursing diagnoses such as *spiritual distress*, he or she may have a simplistic notion of fixing things. Seldom is there a quick fix for spiritual problems.

Nowhere is this more true than where the patient suffers from despair or from a devastating life transition. These spiritual crises are not surmounted without serious spiritual work. And each patient's timetable for overcoming these states (if possible) is his or her own.

SUMMARY

Extreme physical states are likely to bring on spiritual states of anxiety and soul-searching—or as Kubler-Ross notes, bargaining with God. The nurse can be most useful by being a continuing presence through the patient's spiritual struggles rather than by trying to cure them.

Many complexities are involved when a patient is in a state of spiritual anxiety or reaching for spiritual answers. A helpful nurse must be able to discuss spiritual matters without inserting his or her own spiritual goals or religious preferences. Some nurses are very good at being there with such a patient, recognizing that the ultimate path is the patient's, not the nurse's.

Other nurses are unable to keep their own spiritual goals separate from the patient's journey, and this invariably creates difficulties for both the patient and the nurse. Spiritual immaturity on the part of the nurse invariably creates problems. Yet, if the relationship works, the nurse can be an invaluable companion with the patient as he or she resolves his or her spiritual problems and sets his or her new pathway.

REFERENCES

Kierkegaard, S. (1954). *Fear and trembling: The sickness unto death.* New York: Doubleday Anchor Book.

Morse, M. (with Perry, P.) (1994). *Parting visions: Uses and meanings of pre-death, psychic, and spiritual experiences.* New York: Harper Paperbacks.

Morse, M. (with Perry, P.) (1990). *Closer to the light.* New York: Villard Books.

Selder, F. E. (1989). Life transition theory: Resolving uncertainty. *Nursing and Health Care, 10*(8l), 436–440, 449–451.

Selder, F. E. (2010). Personal correspondence.

Schmitt, F. E. (Selder). (1982). *The structure of a life transition following a spinal cord injury.* Unpublished doctoral dissertation, University of Illinois at the Medical Center, Chicago, IL.

BIBLIOGRAPHY

Hawking, S. (1990). *A brief history of time.* New York: Bantam Books.

Kubler-Ross, E. (1969). *On death and dying.* New York: Macmillan.

Kubler-Ross, E. (1975). *Death: The final stage of growth.* Englewood Cliffs, NJ: Prentice Hall.

Kubler-Ross, E. (1997). *The wheel of life: A memoir of living and dying.* New York: Scribner.

CHAPTER 12

Spirituality Versus Humanism

This book has focused on spirituality and has differentiated spirituality from religion, but we have not yet differentiated it from basic humanism. Yet we have at times contrasted spirituality with humanism without defining the latter. We'll correct that omission here. How is spirituality different from basic humanism? Indeed, is the difference enough to matter when delivering nursing care?

Spirituality comes in many forms. As both Fowler (1981) and Peck (1993) note (Chapter 2), it ranges from a simple faith, with ritual and a faith community, all the way to personal mystic encounters with the Divine. Fowler's Stage Two (*mythic-literal*) represents the beginning of this development, with unreflective acceptance of a faith community and a belief structure. Peck's Stage Two (*formal-institutional*) illustrates the same beginning attachment to an institution and its rituals.

Fowler's Stage Six represents the final stage (*universalizing faith*), and it is a transcendent state in which people sense an ultimate environment that is inclusive of all being. Peck's final Stage Four is labeled *mystical/communal* and is similar, including people who reach that ultimate stage of mystery.

Hence, both these developmental spiritual models end in a transcendent state in which there is some mystic experiencing of the Divine. Those who reach an advanced state of faith, in a sense, become one with the meaning they have sought through deepening faith. This is perhaps the greatest difference between spirituality and humanism. Spirituality in both models is mystic in its final state: Humanism denies this possibility and is based on human reason.

HUMANISM

Both spirituality and humanism have a sense of the moral, but spirituality relates, as James (1997) said, to men "so far as they apprehend themselves to stand in relation to whatever they may consider the divine" (p. 43). In contrast, humanism is a philosophy that claims an ethical stance that is related not to the Divine (however defined) but to rationality. As Carl Sagan (1980) said, "The Cosmos is all that is or ever was or ever will be" (p. 1).

Humanism is a position that focuses on human dignity and contrasts with any notion of the supernatural or the Divine, that is, any philosophic system that arises from a source other than reason. Many atheists and agnostics claim to be humanists. Essentially, this movement grew up as a countervailing force against religious powers that were not only repressive but also seen as lacking any relationship to the growing body of scientific knowledge. Since the 19th century, humanism has been associated with anticlericalism, focusing on human rights and separating church and state.

As with almost any human endeavor, there are different groups that give humanism slightly different twists, but most hold to two basic principles: *science* and *compassion*.

Science and the scientific method (which includes the primacy of reason) is the humanistic method of learning about reality. This method, humanists say, has given no proof of a God or of anything above and beyond humanity. Human life, and indeed the cosmos, is an accident. In a sense, one might say that humanism makes science its God. In doing so, however, the humanist is vulnerable to forgetting that science itself is neutral concerning values. The same scientific knowledge can be used for good or evil, as we have seen time and again in human history. Certainly, there have been eras and places where science has been used toward racist/genocidal ends, for example.

This belief in science is usually combined with a sense of empathy or compassion for other human beings. These two beliefs are associated with a conviction that we have only the present life and no other lives and no other form of continued existence. Humanists would simply call this realism, that is, that humans only live one life and must optimize on it for themselves and for the world. As so many commercials say, *you only go around once.* Indeed, we might add this as an absolutism of humanism.

Hence, in this one lifetime, one should make decisions about right and wrong according to the common good. In other words, in the realm of values, humanism has much to do with ethics (see Chapter 7) and nothing to do with spirituality or religion.

This is not to say that spirituality ignores ethics but merely to say that spirituality deals first and foremost with divine meaning rather than ethical rights, wrongs, and duties. Humanism deals with what is human, whereas spirituality seeks that which is beyond mere human existence. Essentially, the difference here is the *reason versus faith* argument, or one might cast it as the *reason versus revelation* argument. Empathy and science are the two basic principles on which humanism rests.

Humanism values human beings without accepting the notion that one must place that value on faith in something beyond humanity itself. Humanism centers on human values but, unlike spirituality or religion, sees that the individual's own worth needs nothing else to validate it.

One might, as illustration, compare Maslow's (1970, 1971) stage of self-actualization with his Being values. Being values reach beyond the person himself; they give a sense of something greater than the person having the peak experience. In contrast, self-actualization can be seen as a sense of great satisfaction derived through making the most of one's human abilities.

There are challenges to humanism (as is true for any philosophy). The first is that it normally places human beings outside the scope of connectedness with existence (where the connectedness includes a notion of God or Source). Man is the focus in most humanism and nothing else.

In contrast, Sagan (1980) shows a humanistic source of connectedness:

> But science has found not only that the universe has a reeling and ecstatic grandeur, not only that it is accessible to human understanding, but also that we are, in a very real and profound sense, a part of that Cosmos, born from it, our fate deeply connected with it. (p. xvi)

Additionally, each human being is separate unto himself in that there is no teleologic principle at work; humanity is not heading toward some preordained destiny. Along with this philosophy comes the notion that there are no absolute truths. Humanism allows the values of science and compassion and usually claims no other dictates. However, we'll find a few hidden dictates along the way. The main claim is an assertion that even science changes over time.

Humanism rejects any religious claims of absolute knowledge and privilege. Today, of course, we are struggling against many repressive tendencies from religious groups that think they have the *only answers*. Absolute truth is always scary, and it is frequently bound to a book that is seen as divinely inspired, holy, and absolutely true. Often, however, such books are all too easily interpreted to suit the goals of their human leaders. Although some will see this refusal to accept absolutes as a limitation leading to ultimate relativism, others will see it as an advantage—one that incidentally aims at religious dictates.

One positive feature of humanism is that it asserts faith in man's ability to scientifically determine the truth or falsity of issues. Because humanism developed at the end of the middle ages, this sense of a renaissance in learning was in keeping with that era.

At present, there are many forms of humanism, including one that links humanistic values with Christianity and others that follow formal traditions much like religious services. Today, many Unitarian–Universalist congregations and Ethical Culture societies describe themselves as humanists.

However, many humanists see their stance simply as a personal philosophy, and people label themselves with more or less knowledge of the traditional meaning of the word *humanism*.

Humanists regard the universe as self-existing and not created. Sagan (1980) again presents this notion:

> In many cultures it is customary to answer that God created the universe out of nothing . . . to pursue the question, we must of course ask next where God comes from . . . why not save a step and decide that the origin of the universe is an unanswerable question. If we say that God has always existed, why not save a step and conclude that the universe has always existed? (p. 212)

Humanism asserts that man has emerged as a result of a continuous process of random movement in this universe. One might say that the human being is the product of accidental molecular collisions. Therefore, there is no plan or intention for life and no super intelligence to set such a plan. Life can have a meaning but only if human beings assign it.

Humanism asserts that the universe depicted by modern science outdates any spiritual or cosmically ordained values. These are dismissed as primitive myths. Humanism claims that intelligent enquiry is the way to assign values. The quest for the good life and the betterment of mankind is the central goal of the human being.

NURSING CARE AND HUMANISM

When a patient identifies himself or herself as a humanist, in one sense, that is like someone saying that he or she is very spiritual but not religious. In other words, it doesn't give one much sense of exactly what the person means by that term. It does allow one to assume that the person is saying that he or she holds many values for human beings.

When one chooses to label oneself as a humanist rather than an atheist, it usually indicates a strong sense of moral values. More commonly, when people identify themselves as humanists, they are simply saying that they hold many values for human life. Although the label atheism is negative in that it states what they do *not* believe, humanism is positive in that it indicates what people *do* believe.

When nurses wonder how to relate to humanists, the answer is not difficult. Recall that in Chapter 9, we concluded that some nursing therapies for spiritual needs and queries were very much similar to psychological counseling. These approaches often work very well when dealing with humanists.

The nurse should be careful not to insert religious or spiritual values of his or her own in conversations with such a patient—certainly not in a manner suggestive of proselytizing or criticism. Remember that the patient may hold humanist values just the way others hold religious or spiritual values. The nurse must respect those values.

So essentially, the nurse meets the needs of the humanist just as he or she would meet the needs of someone who professes to be spiritual without further identifying that term, namely by respecting the beliefs to which they give evidence.

SUMMARY

Occasionally, a nurse may be faced with a patient who identifies himself or herself as a humanist. This probably means that the patient shares many values in common with a person who holds spiritual values. Certainly, both groups hold similar beliefs concerning the value of human beings. The values of the humanist, however, do not include a belief in a God or in higher meaning than that associated with the human being. If there is a God in humanism, it is the God of reason.

The beliefs of humanist patients should be honored just as a nurse would honor the values of a religious or spiritual person. If these patients express doubts or concerns about their philosophy, the nurse can usually address these concerns by applying psychological approaches.

REFERENCES

James, W. (1997). *The varieties of religious experience.* New York: Simon & Schuster (A Touchstone Book).

Sagan, C. (1980). *Cosmos.* New York: Ballantine Books.

BIBLIOGRAPHY

Fowler, J. W. (1981). *Stages of faith: The psychology of human development and the quest for meaning.* San Francisco: HarperSanFrancisco.

Maslow, A. H. (1970). *Motivation and personality* (2nd ed.). New York: Harper and Row.

Maslow, A. H. (1971). *The farther reaches of human nature* (2nd ed.). New York: Viking Press.

Peck, M. S. (1993). *Further along the road less traveled: The unending journey toward spiritual growth.* New York: Simon & Schuster.

CHAPTER 13

Conclusions

As I have said all along, it is difficult to draw specific conclusions that hold for all cases when it comes to the relationship between spirituality and nursing. When it comes to conclusions, we can't really summarize any set of directions for the reader. But what we can summarize are some of the chief obstacles that stand in the way of these relationships, as well as some of the hallmarks that have occurred along the way.

Spirituality has a long association with nursing, probably greatest in early organizing eras when spirituality may have been a great part of what could be offered. Indeed, nursing was originally charged to take care of body, mind, and soul.

In early times, probably from the Knights Templar onward, spirituality usually took the form of religion, especially at times when most countries were dominated by a single religion. And many of these religions were some form of monotheism. Monotheism, alas, tends to bring with it a desire to do away with all other religions. Monotheistic intolerance has lasted many centuries even into our own lifetimes. Indeed, monotheistic zeal is still responsible for much killing and mayhem today as every reader knows.

Western civilization is unique in its tolerance of many religions existing side-by-side. For similar tolerance, one must go back to the Roman and Greek eras of multiple gods where one more deity could easily be integrated into any pantheon.

Beginning in the era of the Knights Templar, patients knew they were in religious institutions, most often in one of their own faith. The perspectives of nurses and the patients on religion were from the same sources. If the nurse read to the patient, it was from a Bible or other holy book with which they both were familiar. If the patient was not of the same religion as the institution where he was being tended, he expected a certain amount of proselytizing to come his way.

In early times, most nurses were religious brothers, nuns, or deaconesses. Again, this pattern is still in existence, despite nursing becoming a secular profession. But the historical association between nursing and spirituality/religion has never totally disappeared.

Nevertheless, as nursing professionalized, the identification of its role changed from looking at the patient as body-mind-soul to seeing him as bio-psycho-social man (or some similar list of components eliminating soul and/or spirituality). Nursing aimed for the scientific arm of its duality: art and science.

However, the connection of spirituality and nursing never totally died out. It was certainly present in early nursing theories where it continues today. In addition to the theories reviewed in Chapter 6, we might add as illustration, theories by Jean Watson (2004), Ina Longway (1960), Rosemary Donley (1991), and Joyce Travelbee (1971). Additionally, holistic nursing (e.g., Barbara Dossey, editor [1997]) also evolved and reinforced links with spirituality because spirituality was seen as a part of the whole person.

As to spiritual dimensions, it is interesting to compare two professions: nursing and psychoanalysis. Despite years of generally ignoring spirituality, nursing has never called spirituality an illusion. Psychoanalysis, in contrast, after the lead of Freud, has, on the whole, supported an atheistic position, which colors many of its psychoanalytic models. Again, these are generalities, and there are exceptions, such as the Association for Spirituality and Psychotherapy—a small but significant backlash to psychoanalytic atheism.

In addition to the ongoing links between nursing and spirituality, there has been an upswing in connections in recent years. Once again, we see accrediting agencies pushing spiritual roles for nurses, as well as similar actions by groups constructing nursing diagnoses.

What these new linkages (demands in some cases) have done is to make us revisit the relationship between nursing and spirituality. And, I might mention, this is occurring in an era when there are equal demands that nursing identify all its tasks in outcome objectives.

The problem this brings, as many chapters in this book have indicated, is that spiritual objectives are not accomplished overnight, except, perhaps for a few rash religious conversions. Where outcome objectives demand deadlines, spiritual objectives often can't measure up. Sometimes nurses solve this, as we have said, by trivializing spiritual outcomes.

Another problem is that spiritual journeys are often initiated by illness and the journeys are not only long but also troubling and self-absorbing. Yet nurses have been trained to stop anything that is painful. Again, this encourages nurses to intervene in the patient's spiritual deliberations, substituting a health-related goal for a spiritual one. Once again we see the pattern of trivializing the patient's search for spiritual meaning.

Obviously, some nurses deal beautifully with spiritual issues, so these comments deal only with a portion of nurses. Yet these cases are the ones that come to the attention of nurse managers. Indeed, I've seen the husband (then a patient) of a well-known nurse theorist, expel a young nurse out of ICU when she tried to provide spiritual counseling. Of course, management-by-exception dictates that only the negative examples, such as this one, are noticed.

The next problem is the spiritually immature nurse who does not recognize his/her limitations. The above example typifies that problem, and the nurse herself in this case, never understood the patient's action. Immaturities also account for most of the proselytizing that goes on—something no patient should have to face when ill.

I think, however, that the problems I have seen most often in this respect occur when a nurse at James Fowler's (1981) Stage Three, synthetic-conventional faith, confronts a patients in Fowler's Stage Four, individuated-reflective faith. You may recall from Chapter 2 that Stage Three involves a very religious person who has committed to a faith with fervor but almost no thought. Stage Four, on the other hand, is the more advanced stage where a patient begins to ask, what is it all about? And this stage frequently begins with a rejection of a former religion that doesn't, at the moment, have any meaning for the patient.

At this stage, we may have a *religious* nurse who sees a patient who is falling away from his faith. From the nurse's perspective, it is impossible to understand that the patient is actually ahead of the nurse and is groping for understanding. So this nurse attempts to get the patient back to where he or she was, namely the nurse's Stage Three. The nurse cannot in his or her spiritual immaturity understand that the patient's rebellion is further advanced, and if the nurse is faced with a directive, such as to treat spiritual distress, the reader can see what will happen. If the nurse succeeds, he or she has squelched the patient's spiritual journey; if the nurse fails, he or she has created an unnecessary conflict with the patient.

For those who prefer M. Scott Peck's (1993) simpler developmental stages, the condition still holds. The same interpretation could be made if the nurse was at Peck's Stage Two, formal-institutional, whereas the patient was at Stage Three, skeptic-individual.

Another great concern is the disconnect where nursing doesn't prepare nurses for spiritual challenges yet expects them to provide spiritual counseling. We typically present little spiritual content in nursing curricula and almost no inculcation that would build spiritual values in the nurse. Yet we write objectives that expect these services from them. Any way one looks at it, we are relying on previous spiritual values that the nurse brings to nursing from other sources in his or her life. It's as if we asked a nurse to do a midwife's job without ever having observed a delivery.

An additional concern is the confusing of spirituality and religion. Many research studies are invalidated by this error, that is, failing to differentiate terms. The study of spirituality often is attempted with quantitative tools when spirituality is a conceptual value. This is not always possible (although it may be used with structural studies of large groups of people). Fowler's study, for example, does this. But for every study that properly applies quantitative tools to spiritual enquiry, there are many studies that are misleading because of faulty research designs.

Yet after all these problems, the greatest problem is the existential dilemma. Whether we like it or not, patients are likely to present spiritual problems to nurses. Nurses are there, patients get to know them, to think of them as experts, albeit in other areas. The sense of authority carries over. The nurse is the one to whom the dilemmas are presented. And often, the only resource available is that nurse.

SUMMARY

What can we say to summarize? Obviously, the more exposure nurses have to spiritual content and spiritual role models, the better. Some institutions do a lot of in-service education with case presentations focusing on spiritual problems. This is wonderful because schools of nursing face the problem of cramming a lot of information into a short period of time. And this tends to further shortchange the study of so-called soft subjects such as spirituality. As technology continues to expand, we can only expect this problem to accelerate.

One ever-present advantage for nurses is that, whereas they don't share a broken leg with a patient, the nurse often shares some vestige of spirituality. So in a sense, many nurses can call upon a personal sense of spirituality when a patient poses questions. More challenging, an agnostic nurse may be drawn into the patient's own sense of not knowing. This ignores those nurses who are atheists, often those who most value the scientific aspect of nursing. They may have little to draw upon (or even negative attitudes) when the patient poses spiritual questions. We must assume that personal philosophies enter nurse–patient relationships when nurses have nothing else to call on.

Nurses have always been expected to take up the slack when professionals from other disciplines are not in attendance. For emergencies, nurses become respiratory therapists, physicians, and nutritionists. And they also become spiritual experts when patients feel the need for immediate answers. One may criticize these steps into lesser known domains, but they all come back to the existential fact of the nurse being there. Ironically, this takes us to perhaps the nurse's best role in patients' spiritual dilemmas: just being there, listening intently, and not rushing off because the patient's questions (in the nurse's mind) don't have immediate answers.

This is pretty much where we end up with spirituality. The nurse assumes this task, ready or not, if he or she is there when it is an immediate patient need. Because dealing with spirituality cannot be avoided (at least not in all cases), one can encourage nurses to take advantage of any learning opportunity (experiential or reading) that presents itself.

A sensitivity to the spiritual is an attitude that can't be taught, but fortunately, many nurses have such a sensitivity. Indeed, they may have been drawn to nursing by this temperament.

BIBLIOGRAPHY

Donley, R. (1991). Spiritual dimensions of health care: Nursing's mission. *Nursing & Health Care, 12*(4), 178–183.

Dossey, B. M. (Ed.). (1997). *Core curriculum for holistic nursing.* Gaithersburg, MD: Aspen Publication.

Fowler, J. W. (1981). *Stages of faith: The psychology of human development and the quest for meaning.* San Francisco: HarperSanFrancisco.

Longway, I. (1960). Toward a philosophy of nursing. *Journal of Adventist Education, 32*(3), 20–27.

Peck, M. S. (1993). *Further along the road less traveled: The unending journey toward spiritual growth.* New York: Simon & Schuster.

Travelbee, J. (1971). *Interpersonal aspects of nursing.* Philadelphia: F. A. Davis.

Watson, J. (2004). *Caring science as sacred science.* Philadelphia: F. A. Davis.

Coda

When the first and second editions of this book were published, I had many protests from readers stating that, after finishing the whole book, they had no idea of my own notion of spirituality. This was a valid criticism because I had tried very hard to keep my own views out of it. But rather than face these complaints again, I'm attaching this very brief view of my own sense of the spiritual.

My formulation is not a very original one, except perhaps for the fact that it flows from experience not cognition and tends to be confirmed by my clients' experiences in altered states of consciousness, particularly during hypnotic regression sessions. The simplest axiom in my world might be *All is one* and that everything flows from a single *Source*. I like this term better than the *God* term because for me, the latter feels like a personal name. I perceive of Source more like a flowing intelligent river than a superhero.

For me, everything comes from Source, the distribution possibly starting with the Big Bang. With this notion, man is a part of Source, not something created separately by Source. The same is true for every blade of grass. *All is one*. I envision human beings as existing at the outer fringe of Source so to speak, where matter has much more density than it has elsewhere.

I don't know if we dwell in the place heaviest with matter, but I know it is heavy enough to be a burden. I also credit this heavy matter for creating the structures we use to make sense of things, namely time and space. Elsewhere it isn't like that, and in many instances, things tend to happen *all at once*. This, of course plays havoc with our sense of causality. Similar to time and space, causality is a major way in which we interpret reality here.

I think that different states of consciousness give us different perceptions of reality. Hence, our perceptions are created by our perceptual tools, the ones created by our bodily sensory input channels. And different entities have different inputs. And these different states of perception are like looking at the same reality through different lenses. That doesn't mean that one perception is correct and another wrong, although some may be clearer pictures than others in various respects. I'm reminded that, even here, we accept the fact that dogs have a greater sense of smell than humans. Indeed, we use them for purposes that require this asset. And we accept their enhanced smell as valid because we see that it consistently reveals a meaningful reality, albeit a different one than human smell perceptions. Perception doesn't equal reality; perception equals a selected view of reality.

Just as the dogs have a different perception from us, I think there are many different levels of reality, probably with entities experiencing their own unique perceptions. And some of us occasionally get into an enhanced perceptual state where we temporarily see through a different set of perceptual organs. Some of us get enough touches of these alternate existences to see what they reveal, and we come to recognize that these states exist in some sense although they are not native to our normal perceptions.

In a global sense, however, it seems to me that things seem to function in hierarchies, although again this may be a human perception. Still, I'll use that image, and through it I see, farther up the line, so to speak, as one example, that the experience of *Cosmic Consciousness* conveys a reality quite different than the one we experience in this material universe.

In cosmic consciousness, everything that is, is all happening at the same time. Except that there really isn't any time at all, so it doesn't even make sense to say, *at the same time*. When one has this experience, one has no sense of being a separate self: *all is one*.

In essence, different realities call on different sense perceptions and there are many different realities. Within this basic construct, I have always seen various religions and spiritual interpretations as consisting in different vibrations, often represented by different colors, often psychedelic, usually quite beautiful. It seems to me that most of these visual images of religions and spiritual states are similar to spokes on a wheel, all leading to the same center. Yes, there are some spokes that have shred apart or twisted off leading nowhere. Some spokes are very broad carrying numerous travelers and some are so thin as to carry a single individual. And that's all okay.

So, no, I don't follow any religion. My notions don't quite fit any church liturgy I've heard. But then I'm drawn to experiences, not dogma. I'm aware that some religions/spiritual philosophies come close, but often I find that members of these groups hold social constraints that just don't fit with my psyche.

Although I find that my beliefs stem from experience, I might add that I have never used drugs to foster experiences. I've had too many patients who went that route, opening doors that they were unprepared to handle, often unable to close them once these doors were opened.

If anyone asks me, I suggest meditation as the best route to knowledge. Yet, I've never been a meditator myself. In any case, I've always found things to be much more complicated than we usually imagine—more dimensions than just time and space, more *places* than just this particular world or solar system.

I don't use the term, *place*, in the same sense as an astronaut, however, because the places to which I refer may be located atop each other. These alternate existences may not be spatial at all. Indeed, they may be right here, just functioning at a different vibratory level, making them normally not perceivable with our available perceptual tools. I think most of us now and then slip across the veil between worlds, even if only a few times in a lifetime, even if only in dreams.

Any sense of comfort in the known has never lasted too long for me. There is always a sense of a bigger reality out there. I am often reminded of the quantum physics theory of Hugh Everett, John Wheeler, and Neill Graham who suggest that the wave function in physics does not just produce one alternative with the other potential outcomes just disappearing. Instead, they propose that all possibilities come into existence in different worlds that coexist with ours.

Many of us may have moments when we accidentally slip into one of those alternate worlds. At times, I think the difference between sanity and insanity is knowing when this happens and knowing when you're back on familiar turf. I've had clients over the years, usually labeled as schizophrenic, who couldn't tell the difference.

For a simple example: I was once in a major hospital in New York City, in an elevator that stopped at the eighth floor where a very attractive female physician stepped in. I looked at her legs and asked, "Oh, do you still do ballet?" She answered, "I don't have much time now. But how did you know?" I proceeded to tell her in detail how the formation of all her leg muscles ruled out any other explanation. And then the elevator stopped, she smiled and got out.

I was terribly glad she got out right then because at exactly that moment, all my knowledge of ballet and muscle formation went right out of my mind. Ballet is something I know almost nothing about in this particular life. For a moment, I had slipped into a different life line along a different wave function—or at least that was the first notion that came to my mind.

Or, I think of a friend who found a delightful hidden room in her attic. But the next time she visited, it no longer existed. A temporary trip to another reality?

With regression clients, I often think that some of the past lives they recount may have occurred in coexistent realities. And I think of the researchers hunting for *proof* that the experiences of reincarnation were real (e.g., old records, historical documents). I think they will only find this proof if the lives they research happened to have been lived in this particular wave function. Alternately, the lives clients envision may indeed be mental and not have occurred in relation to any wave function.

So is that a perspective on the reality that undergirds my sense of the spiritual? It's at least a perception that starts in mind, not in matter, in unfolding rather than pure accident.

For many of us, it's difficult to internalize some of the characteristics of reality revealed by quantum mechanics and newer ideas of physics. That's because so much of our everyday world can be explained on Newtonian physics. It's a simpler world, one we can grasp with less fear, a world in which we are more at home. A world in which we have more control—and that feels safer. Yet many alternate states come closer to images from a quantum physics outlook. And, indeed, it is strange to occasionally find oneself existing in these very different states.

We all have our own versions, our own notions of the world in which we live (and beyond). We attempt to indoctrinate our children into our particular views, although it is unlikely that any two people have exactly the same viewpoint.

Within the world where we happen to find ourselves, it seems to me that most of us are struggling to grow toward more understanding, more comfort in the larger scene—however large that view is for the individual. It seems to me that we pick up strands of understanding as we go.

I see that same urge to grow toward greater understanding and greater being in my clients. I find interesting commonalities among them. For example, the experiences they have under regression are similar regardless of whether they go into the experience believing in the concept of alternate lives. It reminds me of the similarity of near-death encounters, again, where the patient's prior beliefs don't seem to entirely control the experience.

Because, in my view, *all is one*, it certainly makes no sense to treat each other as if we were separate beings. So kindness and sensitivity are more or less just common sense and even self-interest. And so much cruelty in the world seems to depend on a notion that we are separate and different. That's a very short version of the beliefs that touch on my sense of the spiritual. I realize that these beliefs are different than those promulgated in most religions popular in this nation, particularly that human beings are not seen as entities created by God. Yet I'm aware that my own perception of man as *part* of God (Source in my terms) is far from unusual.

I hope that those small glimpses help any curious reader who wants to know from where my notion of the spiritual comes. It's possible that some of these ideas are *farther out* than most of the ideas in this book. And that seems logical to me because many readers have a different perspective than mine. One advantage of focusing on spirituality rather than religion is that people share more in common in this dimension. Ultimately, whatever beliefs undergird our sense of spirit, most of us have the same sense of touching the divine, of linking to the greatest meaning. Does it matter if the details are different?

Index

A

Alcoholic Anonymous (AA)
  programs, 41
altered states of consciousness
  in shamanism, 37
  use of, 41
amygdala, 29
anima, 58
animus, 58
archetype, 58
association areas of brain, 39–40
attention association area, 40
auditory driving, 37, 44
  drumbeat of, 44
aural layers, 110
ayahuasca, 43

B

Benson, Herbert, 49–50
blaming, 140–143
brain
  association areas of, 39–40
  and auditory driving, 44
  and contemplative acts, 36–38
  and cosmic consciousness, 40
  and hemisync methods, 44
  and meditation, 36, 38–40
  and mind, 50–51
  and near-death experiences
    (NDEs), 30–31
  and spirituality, 27–44
  and substance abuse, 40–44
  and temporal-limbic system,
    28–30
  wave frequencies of, 38

C

Cayce, Edgar, 108
chakra energy vortices, 113–114
channeling, 108
chaotic/antisocial stage, 21
cognitive behavioral therapy (CBT),
  55, 59–60
cognitive therapy (CT), 55, 59–60
collective unconsciousness, 58
communities and organizations
  developmental models for, 14–18
conjunctive faith, 20
contemplation, 22, 36–38
  See also meditation
context versus spirituality,
  129, 135–137
cosmic consciousness and
  meditation, 40

D

date rape drug, 42
death and dying. *See* dying
  and death
deliriants, 42
depersonalization, 29
derealization, 29
despair, 139, 148–149
disability, 139, 146–148
discursive meditation, 36
dissociatives, 42
dreamy states, 30
drive theory, 55–56
dying and death, 139, 143
  and hospice movement, 143–144
  predeath experiences, 144–145